Microbial diseases of occupations, sports and recreations

C.H. Collins
MBE, DSc, FRCPath, FIBiol
Senior Visiting Research Fellow, Department of Microbiology, National Heart and Lung Institute, Imperial College of Science, Technology and Medicine, University of London

T.C. Aw
MB BS, MSc, PhD, FRCPC, FRCP, FFOM
Senior Lecturer in Occupational Medicine, Institute of Occupational Health, University of Birmingham

J.M. Grange
MD, MSc
Director, Department of Microbiology, National Heart and Lung Institute, Imperial College of Science, Technology and Medicine, University of London

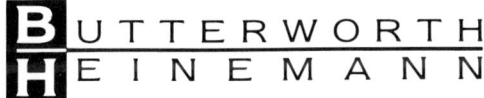

BUTTERWORTH
HEINEMANN

Butterworth-Heinemann
Linacre House, Jordan Hill, Oxford OX2 8DP
A division of Reed Educational and Professional Publishing Ltd

$\mathcal{R}$ A member of the Reed Elsevier plc group

OXFORD   BOSTON   JOHANNESBURG
MELBOURNE   NEW DELHI   SINGAPORE

First published 1997
© Reed Educational and Professional Publishing Ltd 1997

British Library Cataloguing in Publication Data

A catalogue record for this book is available from the British Library.

Library of Congress Cataloguing in Publication Data

A catalogue record for this book is available from the Library of Congress.

ISBN 0 7506 2183 4

Printed and bound in Great Britain by The University Press, Cambridge

Contents

Foreword

Diseases associated with work have been prevalent since humans abandoned the hunter-gatherer lifestyle in favour of specific occupations. As a specialty, occupational health has been recognized for less than a century but it is only in the past few decades that books have appeared which are dedicated to the subject. In more recent times, certain books have concentrated on specific aspects of the subject—notably lung disorders, skin diseases and cancer. To date there has been no text devoted to microbial diseases of occupations.

Drs Collins, Aw and Grange have now filled the gap. Indeed they have gone further by including infectious diseases associated with sports and recreations. Despite the advances made in antimicrobial therapy, some infectious diseases remain a serious threat to life. A disproportionate number of these are associated with occupations and thus a book concentrating on this subject is timely.

The authors are to be congratulated on providing an authoritative volume for those who are responsible for the health care of individuals who could become infected in the course of their work or their recreation.

J. Malcolm Harrington, CBE

Preface

Courses of instruction for candidates who are studying for qualifications in occupational medicine, hygiene and nursing necessarily include microbial diseases and the microbial hazards of occupations. Information on these is scattered widely through books and papers in medical, microbiological and public health journals. We have attempted to bring them all together under one cover and hope that the resulting text will also be of value to qualified practitioners as well as to staff who work in allied areas. We have arranged the text so that readers may refer to the sources of pathogenic and allergenic micro-organisms, occupations and activities and/or specific diseases, according to the problems that present themselves and then proceed to the relevant investigations, methods of control and worker/participant protection.

C.H. Collins
T.C. Aw
J.M. Grange

1 Historical perspective: prescribed, reportable and notifiable microbial diseases

Hippocrates recommended that physicians consider their patients' occupations as part of their examinations. No further evidence of medical interest in the trades or professions of the sick was evinced until Bernardino Ramazzini (1713) published a treatise entitled *De Morbis Artificum Diatriba* which is recognized as the earliest work on occupational diseases. Among various diseases that affected miners and other manual workers he included a description of an affliction of cereal workers, now recognized as farmer's lung, a form of extrinsic allergic alveolitis caused by thermophilic actinomycetes. In addition, his observations on the diseases of cesspit workers indicate that some of them may well have been occupationally acquired infections.

For several centuries workers accepted that disease was the price they had to pay for the privilege of earning their daily bread. It was not until the nineteenth century, and then in the face of much opposition, that some legislation for the protection of workers was introduced. Even then the earliest, the *Health and Morals of Apprentices Act 1802*, was more concerned with the morals of workers than with their health, although some standards of ventilation and cleanliness were included. In the UK, from 1819 until well into the twentieth century a series of factories acts and factory and workshop acts, leading to the formation of the Factory Inspectorate, went some way towards promoting the health and well-being of the workers. Most of the legislation, however, was concerned with injuries rather than with disease. From the point of view of occupational medicine an important step was made in 1898 when the Medical Branch of the Inspectorate was introduced. This was reorganized as the Employment Medical Advisory Service when the *Health and Safety at Work, etc. Act 1974* was implemented.

The history of microbial-associated occupational diseases before the acceptance, in the late nineteenth century, of the 'germ theory of disease' is brief indeed and is clouded by the persistence, even into the early twentieth century, of the 'miasma versus contagion' controversies. Once microbes had

1

been incriminated as agents of infection, however, primarily as a result of the work of the schools of Pasteur, Koch and their successors, a connection between some of the diseases for which they are responsible and the occupations of the patients was suspected, and in some cases proved. The first of these was probably anthrax and this was the subject of the earliest pieces of legislation about an occupational infection. It became 'notifiable' in 1895 and 15 years later *The Anthrax Order 1910* (since superseded) came into effect. Since then anthrax has been the object of a number of orders and regulations governing the reporting of the disease, disposal of infected animal carcases and the importation of animal hides, hair, wool, bone and other raw materials that might be infected with *Bacillus anthracis* spores.

Prescribed diseases

Over the years other microbial diseases of occupations were recognized. It became clear that some form of compensation should be awarded to workers who contracted diseases, or who became incapacitated, in the course of their employment. In 1946 the *National Insurance (Industrial Injuries) Act* provided for the establishment of the Industrial Injuries Advisory Council (IIAC) which came into effect in July 1948. In the UK, evidence that a disease (microbial or other) is occupationally acquired is considered by the Council. The IIAC may then recommend to the Secretary of State at the Department of Social Security (DSS) that the disease be 'prescribed'. The Secretary of State must be satisfied that (a) the disease is a special risk for the occupation, and (b) the attribution of the disease to the work can be established with reasonable certainty.

In 1981 the IIAC recommended rationalization of the list of occupationally acquired diseases and this was embodied in the *Social Security (Industrial Injuries) (Prescribed Diseases) Regulations 1985*. At present the prescribed 'conditions due to biological agents' (in the context of this book microbial diseases), and the conditions under which they become prescribed (IIAC, 1993) are shown in Table 1.1. Of these diseases anthrax, glanders, ankylostomiasis, *Streptococcus suis* infection and hydatid disease now occur rarely, if at all, in the UK.

A worker who acquires a prescribed disease under the above conditions is eligible to be considered for compensation. Claims must be made to the local offices of the DSS, which provides forms for that purpose. After the forms have been processed the claimant is required to be medically assessed. If the assessors agree that the claimant has a prescribed disease, financial benefits are awarded, depending on the extent of the disability. Under the current procedures there must be at least 14% disability for the benefits to be

Table 1.1 *Prescribed diseases—conditions caused by biological agents*

No. and disease		Type of job: any job involving
B1	Anthrax	Contact with animals infected with anthrax or the handling (including the loading or unloading or transport) of animal products or residues.
B2	Glanders	Contact with equine animals or their carcases.
B3	Infection by leptospira	(a) Work in places which are, or are liable to be, infested by rats, field mice or voles, or other small mammals; or (b) work at dog kennels or the care or handling of dogs; or (c) contact with bovine animals or their meat products or pigs or their meat products.
B4	Ankylostomiasis	Work in or around a mine.
B5	Tuberculosis	Contact with a source of tuberculous infection.
B6	Extrinsic allergic alveolitis (including farmer's lung)	Exposure to moulds or fungal spores or heterologous proteins by reason of their employment in: (a) agriculture, horticulture, forestry, cultivation of edible fungi or malt working; or (b) loading or unloading or handling in storage mouldy vegetable matter or edible fungi; or (c) care for or handling birds; or (d) handling bagasse.
B7	Infection by organisms of the genus *Brucella*	Contact with: (a) animals infected by *Brucella*, or their carcases or parts thereof, or their untreated products; or (b) laboratory specimens or vaccines of, or containing, *Brucella*.
B8	Viral hepatitis	Contact with: (a) human blood or human blood products; or (b) a source of viral hepatitis.
B9	Infection by *Streptococcus suis*	Contact with pigs infected by *Streptococcus suis*, or with the carcases, products or residues of pigs so infected.

(continued)

Table 1.1 (*continued*)

No. and disease		Type of job: any job involving
B10		
(a)	Avian chlamydiosis	Contact with birds infected with *Chlamydia psittaci*, or with the remains or untreated products of such birds.
(b)	Ovine chlamydiosis	Contact with sheep infected with *Chlamydia psittaci*, or with the remains or untreated products of such sheep.
B11	Q fever	Contact with animals, their remains or their untreated products.
B12	Orf	Contact with sheep, goats or with the carcases of sheep or goats.
B13	Hydatidosis	Contact with dogs.

Reproduced from the *Industrial Injuries Advisory Council Periodic Report 1993* (IIAC, 1993). Crown copyright is reproduced with the permission of the Controller of HMSO.

payable. There is also provision for a periodic review of the case in the event that the disease is progressive.

Tables 1.2 and 1.3 show the numbers of cases of prescribed diseases for which assessment for compensation has been made during the period 1986-1993 (infections) and 1983-1992 (allergies).

The National Health Service also has an industrial injuries benefit scheme for its employees.

The Reporting of Injuries, Diseases and Dangerous Occurrences Regulations 1995

Under these regulations ('RIDDOR'), which were revised in 1995, the occurrences which must be reported are grouped under poisonings, skin diseases, lung diseases, infections and other conditions. Employers are required to report these diseases to the Health and Safety Executive (HSE) if they occur in someone employed in a prescribed occupation or work activity (see Table 1.4). This is usually initiated on receipt of a doctor's note indicating that the employee has a specific infection. The onus is on the employers to check if the employee works in a prescribed occupation. If so the case has to be notified. The principle behind reporting is that areas of concern may

Table 1.2 *Prescribed diseases: new cases assessed for disablement 1986–1993*

	1986–87	1987–88	1988–89	1989–90	1990–91	1991–92	1992–93
Anthrax					1		
Leptospirosis	1			2		1	1
Tuberculosis	13	3	5	3	3	3	6
Brucellosis	2		1	2	1	1	2
Viral hepatitis	5	3	1	1	2	4	2
Streptococcus suis	3				1		
Avian chlamydiosis	NA	NA			1		2
Ovine chlamydiosis	NA	NA			1	1	
Q fever	NA	NA			1		
Orf	NA	NA	NA	NA	NA	2	2

NA = not applicable during that period.
Abstracted from *Industrial Injuries Advisory Council Periodic Report 1993* (IIAC, 1993). Crown copyright is reproduced with the permission of the Controller of HMSO.

Table 1.3   *Prescribed diseases: new cases of extrinsic alveolitis, including farmer's lung, and occupational asthma, assessed for disablement, 1983–1992*

	1983	1984	1985	1986	1987	1988	1989	1990	1991	1992
Extrinsic alveolitis	8	4	6	11	8	15	13	7	5	5
Occupational asthma	183	137	166	166	220	223	220	216	293	555

Abstracted from *Industrial Injuries Advisory Council Periodic Report 1993* (IIAC, 1993). Crown copyright is reproduced with the permission of the Controller of HMSO.

be identified by the HSE and appropriate action taken. Reports must be made on officially approved forms (Form F2508A for disease; Form F2508B for accidents). Microbial diseases occurring on farms, in horticulture or forestry must be reported to the HSE Agricultural Inspectorate: those that occur in factories, offices and other premises to the HSE Factory Inspectorate. Addresses and telephone numbers of HSE Inspectorates may be found in local telephone directories and are listed in a guide to the regulations (HSE, 1986).

The RIDDOR list of microbial diseases, made reportable in 1995, is all embracing (Table 1.4).

In addition to the infections, etc. in Table 1.4, all infections notifiable under the *Public Health (Control of Diseases) Act, 1984* and the *Public Health*

Table 1.4   *Infections, etc. due to biological agents reportable under RIDDOR*

Anthrax	Lyme disease
Brucellosis	Ovine chlamydidosis
Avian chlamydiosis	Rabies
Hepatitis	*Streptococcus suis* infection
Legionellosis	Tetanus
Leptospirosis	Tuberculosis

Work with micro-organisms; work with live or dead human beings in the course of providing any treatment or service or in conducting any investigation involving exposure to blood or body fluids; work with animals or any potentially infected material derived from above.
Extrinsic alveolitis (including farmer's lung)

(*Infectious Diseases*) *Regulations, 1988* (Table 1.5), and occurring among workers in off-shore workplaces, must be reported under RIDDOR.

HSE publish useful guides to RIDDOR (HSE, 1986) and 'RIDDOR 95' (see Appendix 2).

In recent years it has become apparent that people who engage in various sporting and recreational activities, initially water sports but later various field and 'contact' sports, are also at risk from microbial infections, derived from either the environment in which they enjoy their activities, or from other people during the course of those activities. Such diseases qualify as occupational only when the individual is an employee of the sporting or recreational organization, and cases must also be reported under RIDDOR, although the 'Duty of Care' under the *Health and Safety at Work etc. Act 1974* still applies. By the same token any disease acquired by people who travel abroad in pursuit of their occupations or organized sports may be considered as occupational.

Notifiable infectious diseases

The *Public Health (Control of Diseases) Act, 1984* lists cholera, plague, relapsing fever, smallpox and typhus as 'notifiable diseases'. The *Public Health (Infectious Diseases) Regulations 1988* require that a number of other infectious diseases must also be notified by the attending physician to the local Consultant for Communicable Disease Control. The current list, which includes both 'notifiable diseases' and 'diseases which are required to be notified', applicable in England and Wales, is shown in Table 1.5. In Scotland the list includes other diseases; these are given in the footnote to Table 1.5. These lists are included here because some of the diseases are prescribed and also reportable under RIDDOR.

Actions to be taken in respect of a disease, other than one of the five 'notifiable diseases', are given in Schedule 1 of the *Public Health (Infectious Diseases) Regulations 1988.*

It will be seen that there is a considerable overlap in the lists of prescribed, reportable and notifiable diseases. The reasons for this lie in the different purposes of the three sets of regulations which are administered differently by the Department of Social Security, the Department of Health, and the Health and Safety Executive (Department of Employment) respectively.

Table 1.5   *Statutorily notifiable infectious diseases in England and Wales[1]*

1. Notifiable under the *Public Health (Control of Diseases) Act 1984:*

Cholera	Smallpox
Plague	Typhus
Relapsing fever	

2. Diseases which must be notified under the *Public Health (Control of Disease) Regulations 1988:*

Acute encephalitis	Mumps
Acute poliomyelitis	Ophthalmia neonatorum‡
Anthrax	Paratyphoid fever
Dysentery (amoebic and bacillary)*	Rabies
	Rubella
Food poisoning†	Scarlet fever
Leprosy	Tetanus
Leptospirosis	Tuberculosis
Malaria	Typhoid fever
Measles	Viral haemorrhagic fever
Meningitis	Viral hepatitis
Meningococcal septicaemia (without meningitis)	Whooping cough
	Yellow fever

[1] In Scotland the list includes chickenpox, Lyme disease, membranous croup and toxoplasmosis.
* Dysentery. For purposes of notification, any case with acute symptoms of enteritis, accompanied by the passage of blood or mucus, should be regarded as dysentery.
† Food poisoning. Food poisoning is an illness, other than typhoid, dysentery, etc. (specifically notified as such), caused by the consumption of food or drink.
‡ Ophthalmia neonatorum. For the purpose of notification the expression 'ophthalmia neonatorum' means a purulent discharge from the eyes of an infant, commencing within 21 days from the date of birth.

2 Reservoirs and sources of micro-organisms

Micro-organisms are ubiquitous, occupying and colonizing sites as disparate as arctic ice and volcanic rocks, ocean depths and land deserts. Those that are associated with diseases of occupations and with sports and recreations tend to occur in less extreme conditions. Some micro-organisms live freely in the environment but are able to cause disease in humans and animals. Others have devolved to a total dependence on a living host. Some of the latter may survive in the inanimate environment for long periods but others depend on direct transmission from host to host for their survival (see Chapter 3).

The sites in which micro-organisms are found form reservoirs or sources and may be the natural or man-made environment, animals and human beings themselves. There may be direct contact between these reservoirs and those who acquire the diseases or there may be vehicles or vectors that disperse or transmit the micro-organisms from reservoirs to people. Reservoirs, sources and vehicles are listed below alphabetically rather than in order of importance.

Aerosols and droplet nuclei

Strictly speaking, aerosols are colloidal systems, e.g. mists or fogs, in which the dispersion medium is a gas, e.g. air. They are formed when liquids are mechanically disturbed, e.g when bubbles burst, when liquids are forced through fine jets or when they impinge upon solid surfaces. The more violent the disturbance the more likely the formation of aerosols and the smaller the droplets. Examples of aerosol formation in natural, domestic and industrial circumstances are fast-flowing rivers that are interrupted by solid surface objects, waterfalls, fountains and jets from garden hoses, showers, fire sprinklers, industrial mixers and agitators, humidifiers and air-conditioning cooling towers, and mists from metal-working fluids. Aerosols are also generated by sneezing and coughing and serve as vectors for transmission of respiratory pathogens.

If the liquid contains micro-organisms, these will be present in the aerosol droplets singly, in clumps or attached to inert particles. The larger droplets (>5 μm in diameter) settle rapidly under the influence of gravity. The smaller droplets (<5 μm in diameter) settle slowly but dry rapidly, leaving their microbial contents, known as droplet nuclei, suspended in air. These smaller droplets are little affected by gravity and are moved around by even the smallest of air currents. Aerosols and droplet nuclei are thus vehicles that transfer micro-organisms from site to site and site to person (Collins, 1993). Particles of 5 μm or less are more likely to reach the alveoli of the lung than the larger particles which tend to impinge on the walls of the nose and pharynx, or on the ciliary escalator in the trachea or larger bronchi.

Lacey and Dutkiewicz (1994) have expanded the above definition and use the term 'bioaerosol' to include suspensions in air of any particles of biological origin. Bioaerosols have been implicated in occupational lung diseases and include viruses, bacteria and fungal spores and mycelial fragments, as well as pollens and other particulate plant and animal material.

Air

'Fresh' air contains relatively few micro-organisms. Figures of 10^4 bacteria and 10^3 fungal spores per m^3 are not unusual. But human activities greatly augment these numbers (Crook and Lacey, 1991). Table 2.1 shows concentrations of airborne organisms that have been found in some work environments.

Air-conditioning plant and humidifiers

These are fruitful sources of micro-organisms and endotoxins associated with respiratory diseases (Rylander *et al.*, 1978; Rylander and Haglind, 1984; Waldron, 1990). The cooling towers of air-conditioning plants may be reservoirs of *Legionella* species. *Legionella pneumophila* was responsible for the first recognized outbreak of legionnaires' disease at a hotel in Philadelphia in 1976. This outbreak led to the subsequent isolation and identification of the causative organism. Perhaps this outbreak can be classed as a recreation-related infection as it occurred among members of the American Legion who were attending a convention. *Legionella pneumophila* is a ubiquitous organism, frequently isolated from water systems in hospitals, hotels and office blocks.

Anatomical laboratories

See Animals and Cadavers.

Table 2.1   *Numbers* of airborne micro-organisms found in the air in work environments*

Workplace (reference)	Total bacteria	Gram-negative bacteria	Thermophilic actinomyces	Total fungi	Predominant species
Outdoors (1)	10^4	10^1	10^1	10^3	
MSW† tipping halls (1)	10^4	10^3	10^3	10^5	Aspergillus Penicillium
Pig farms (2)	10^6	—	10^3	10^5	Gram-positive rods, cocci
Mushroom composting picking (3)	10^6 10^3	— —	10^7 10^2	10^5 10^5	Actinomycetes Penicillium Plicaria
Sugar-beet processing (4)	10^5	10^3	10^2	10^3	Leuconostoc Enterobacter
Metal-working fluids (5)	10^6				Pseudomonas

* Numbers = colony-forming units/m³.
† Municipal solid waste.
Adapted from Crook (1991) by permission of *Laboratory News*.
References: (1) Crook and Lacey (1988); (2) Crook *et al.* (1991); (3) Crook and Lacey (1991); (4) Forster *et al.* (1989); (5) Travers Glass *et al.* (1991).

Animals

Zoonoses, i.e. diseases of animals transmissible to humans, are widespread. Over 150 are known world-wide (Danham, 1985) but many of them require arthropod vectors for transmission to humans. Only two such zoonoses that require arthropod vectors, Lyme disease and louping ill (ovine encephalitis), occur among the 30 or so indigenous to the UK. Some zoonoses are genus or species specific. Others, such as infections by *Pasteurella multocida*, affect a wide variety of animals. Some, such as *Mycobacterium bovis*, have a preferred host but many other species may develop transmissible disease. From an occupation-, sport- and recreation-related disease aspect, however, animals may be placed in three general but not exclusive groups; indigenous, exotic and experimental, which may include both indigenous and exotic species. There is a Health and Safety Executive (HSE, 1993c) publication on occupational zoonoses but for detailed accounts of all known zoonoses see Bell *et al.* (1988) and Acha and Szyfres (1989).

Table 2.2   *Zoonoses of indigenous and farmed animals*

Animals	Zoonoses
Birds (caged and falconry)	Ornithosis
Badgers	Tuberculosis; borreliosis
Cats	Cat scratch fever; pasteurellosis; ringworms; toxocariasis; toxoplasmosis
Cattle	Anthrax; brucellosis; leptospirosis; listeriosis; milker's nodules; pasteurellosis; ringworms; tapeworms; tuberculosis; cryptosporidiosis; vesicular stomatitis; mycobacteriosis; salmonellosis (calves)
Deer	Borreliosis (Lyme disease); pasteurellosis; salmonellosis
Dogs	Pasteurellosis; ringworms; salmonellosis; tapeworms; toxocariasis
Ferrets	Pasteurellosis
Field mice	Leptospirosis; hantavirus
Fish	Listeriosis; mycobacteriosis
Goats	Brucellosis; cryptosporidiosis
Horses	Glanders; vesicular stomatitis
Mice	Lymphocytic choriomeningitis
Pigs	Brucellosis; erysipeloid; listeriosis; salmonellosis; tapeworms; pseudorabies; vesicular stomatitis
Poultry	Newcastle disease; pasteurellosis; salmonellosis; psittacosis
Rats	Leptospirosis; pasteurellosis; rat bite fever; salmonellosis; hantavirus infection
Sheep	Anthrax; brucellosis; orf; Q fever; ovine chlamydiosis; enzootic abortion; ringworms
Voles	Leptospirosis; listeriosis; hantavirus

Indigenous animals

Many of these are farmed for human consumption, when abattoirs may also become reservoirs of infection. Some are domestic animals, and a few may be encountered in sporting and recreational activities. Some feral species are also included. Indigenous animals and their associated zoonoses are listed in Table 2.2. Useful references for farm animals are Danham (1985) and Thomas and Joynson (1995).

Table 2.3 *Exotic zoonoses that may be imported*

Zoonosis (causative organism)	Animal reservoir (area)
Relapsing fever*	Rodents, pigs, armadillos (Africa, Asia, Latin America)
Rabies	Dogs
Hydatid disease	Dogs
Leishmaniasis*	Dogs, various wild animals (Africa, Middle East, Asia, South America)
Marburg disease	Green monkeys (Africa)
Lassa fever	Mastomys rats (West and Central Africa)
Plague*	Rats, sussliks, ground squirrels
Rat bite fever	Rats (Far East)
Simian herpes B	Old world monkeys
Trypanosomiasis*	Antelopes, cattle (Africa, South America)
Tularaemia	Rabbits, ground squirrels, rodents, (North America, Scandinavia)
Hantaviruses	Rodents (North America, Northern Europe)
Shigellosis	Monkeys (Old and New World)
Respiratory syncytial virus	Monkeys (Old and New World)

* Arthropod-borne.

Exotic species

These are usually found in zoos, menageries, circuses and pet shops. The list in Table 2.3 includes zoonoses that are acquired by direct contact and those that require arthropod vectors. Although such vectors are not indigenous to the UK, infected travellers may enter the country and their diseases may then qualify as acquired through occupation, sport or recreation.

Experimental and laboratory animals

Several species are used in teaching, medical and other research projects, and also for the diagnosis of communicable diseases. These, and their zoonoses, are shown in Table 2.4. This does not, of course, include deliberate laboratory infections carried out for diagnostic or research purposes.

Table 2.4   *Zoonoses of laboratory and experimental animals*

Animals	Zoonoses
Rodents	Lymphocytic choriomeningitis; salmonellosis; rat bite fevers; leptospirosis; pasteurellosis; erysipeloid; Korean haemorrhagic (Hantaan) fever; ringworms
Cats and dogs	Cat scratch fever; leptospirosis; pasteurellosis; toxocariasis; toxoplasmosis; hydatid disease; ringworms; rabies
Simians	Simian B disease; Marburg disease; rabies; Kyasanur Forest disease; salmonellosis; shigellosis; tuberculosis; respiratory syncytial virus infection; intestinal parasites

Table 2.5 lists the causative agents of some zoonoses that may be acquired during occupational, sporting and recreational activities.

Allergy to laboratory animals (ALA) commonly occurs among animal technicians and attendants. Although most of the allergens are related to dusts, fur, feathers, etc. some may be of a microbial nature (Agrup *et al.*, 1986; HSE, 1990a).

Animal products

Edible products are considered later under Foodstuffs. Non-edible products include skins, hides, hairs and wool; also, bones are used to make bonemeal for fertilizers. Many of these are imported: goat and camel hair from the Middle and Far East and the Indian subcontinent, dry and dry-salted hides from Africa, Asia and Central and South America, bones and bonemeal from almost anywhere. In developing countries these are all important reservoirs of *Bacillus anthracis*, the agent of anthrax. This disease is rare in developed countries because of import restrictions and disinfection requirements. Even in developed countries, however, these products may harbour dermatophyte (ringworm) fungi.

There is current concern about the use, in feeding stuffs, of offal, etc. of animals that have been infected with one of the 'unconventional agents', such as the prions responsible for scrapie and bovine spongiform encephalopathy (BSE). This practice is now illegal. Cross infection of humans has not been proved but the possibilities should be kept under review.

Table 2.5   *Zoonoses—causative organisms*

Anthrax	*Bacillus anthracis*
Brucellosis	*Brucella abortus, B. melitensis, B. suis*
Cat scratch fever	*? Rochalimea* spp
Chagas' disease	*Trypanosoma cruzi*
Erysipeloid	*Erysipelothrix rhusiopathiae*
Giardiasis	*Giardia lamblia*
Glanders	*Pseudomonas mallei*
Hantaan pulmonary syndrome	Hantaviruses
Lassa fever	Lassa fever virus
Leishmaniasis (kala azar)	*Leishmania donovani*
Leptospirosis	*Leptospira interrogans*
Louping ill (ovine encephalitis)	Louping ill virus
Lyme disease	*Borrelia burgdorferi*
Lymphocytic choriomeningitis	LCM virus
Marburg disease	Marburg virus
Milker's nodules	Paravaccinia virus
Mycobacteriosis	*Mycobacterium marinum*
Newcastle disease conjunctivitis	Newcastle disease virus
Orf (contagious pustular dermatitis)	Orf virus
Ornithosis/psittacosis	*Chlamydia psittaci*
Ovine chlamydiosis (enzootic abortion)	*Chlamydia psittaci*
Pasteurellosis	*Pasteurella multocida*
Plague	*Yersinia pestis*
Q fever	*Coxiella burnettii*
Rabies	Rabies virus
Rat bite fever	
USA	*Streptobacillus moniliformis*
Far East	*Spirillum minus*
Relapsing fever (tickborne)	*Borrelia duttoni*
Ringworms	*Trichophyton* spp
(dermatomycoses)	*Microsporum* spp
Salmonellosis	*Salmonella* serotypes
Shigellosis	*Shigella* spp
Simian B disease	Herpesvirus simiae
Tapeworms	*Taenia saginata*
Toxocariasis	*Toxocara canis, T. cati*
Toxoplasmosis	*Toxoplasma gondii*
Trypanosomiasis	*Trypanosoma brucei*
(African sleeping sickness)	*T. rhodesiense*
Tuberculosis	*Mycobacterium tuberculosis,*
	M. bovis
Tularaemia	*Francisella tularensis*
Typhus, murine spotted fever	*Rickettsia mooseri*
	R. rickettsii
Vesicular stomatitis	Vesicular stomatitis virus

Biotechnology

Many different micro-organisms are used in the biotechnology industries and may escape from processes in leaks, spillages and aerosols in spite of the stringent precautions that are taken to 'contain' them (Chapter 10). Very few of these organisms qualify as pathogens—only those that are used to make certain vaccines, therapeutic agents and diagnostic materials. Nevertheless, although the others are incapable of causing infections, they may be associated with other illnesses. Some organisms used in biotechnology, and also some products, associated with respiratory disease are shown in Table 2.6. Some non-infectious diseases associated with the use of micro-organisms in biotechnology are shown in Table 2.7.

There is a potential for the release of endotoxins during large-scale processes with Gram-negative bacilli, e.g. *Escherichia coli* in the manufacture of proteins (Palchak *et al.*, 1988). This may be controlled by engineering methods. Enzymes may also present a problem and workers who are exposed, especially if they suffer from chronic respiratory or skin disorders, should be tested for susceptibility and, if indicated, assigned to other work. There is no

Table 2.6   *Micro-organisms and products used in biotechnology and associated with occupational respiratory disease*

	Process
Organism:	
Aspergillus spp.	Fermentation
Aspergillus niger	Citric acid production
Baculoviruses	Pesticide production
Candida tropicalis	Protein production
Methylophilus methylotrophus	Single cell protein
Methylamonas methanolica	Pharmaceutical production
Pseudomonas aeruginosa	Downstream processing
Product:	
Ampicillin	Antibiotic production
Tetracycline	Antibiotic production
Penicillin	Antibiotic production
Subtilisin	Biological washing powder
Amylase	Enzyme production
Cellulase	Enzyme production

From Bennett (1987). Reproduced by permission of *Laboratory News*.

Table 2.7   *Non-infectious illness associated with biotechnology*

Product/process	Illness
Antibiotics	Haemorrhagic rhinitis, cardiovascular disorders, opportunistic colonization
Brewing	Dermatitis, malt fever
Citric acid production	Asthma, bronchitis
Enzymes	Asthma, conjunctivitis, dermatitis
Endotoxins	Influenza symptoms on inhalation
Fungal fermentations	Asthma, bronchitis
Single cell protein	Allergic responses, asthma, dermatitis

Adapted from Hambleton *et al.* (1992), by permission of the authors and Elsevier Trends journals.
(Data from Duffus and Brown, 1985; Bennet and Norris, 1989).

evidence that risks in biotechnology are any different from those in other kinds of work.

Fears that biotechnologists might accidentally create new and virulent micro-organisms by genetic modification appear to be unfounded (WHO, 1982a; Lieberman *et al.*, 1991). The use of animal cell lines in tissue cultures has aroused some concern because these cells may be infected with organisms such as *Mycoplasma* spp. 'slow viruses', or prions responsible for scrapie and BSE, collectively known as transmissible spongiform encephalopathies (TSEs) (Beale, 1992; Basel Forum on Biosafety, 1993). There is a greater uncertainty in this respect about primary cell lines than about diploid cell lines (Frommer *et al.*, 1993). According to the Advisory Committee on Dangerous Pathogens (HSE, 1994a) there is no evidence of transmission of TSEs to workers.

Blood

Many people, apart from those engaged in healthcare, may accidentally come into contact with human blood during their work or sporting activities. Bloodborne diseases have achieved some prominence in recent years. Of these, the three that seem to pose a real hazard in the UK are hepatitis B, hepatitis C and infection by the human immunodeficiency virus (HIV), which may progress to the acquired immunodeficiency syndrome (AIDS). Contact, even with infected blood, does not necessarily result in transmission of the viruses or development of the diseases. The number of virus particles in the blood in each disease differs, being greatest in hepatitis B, less in hepatitis C and relatively low in HIV infections. The chances of infection from hollow needle injuries where blood is involved seem to be of the order of 1 in 5 for hepatitis B, 1 in 10 for hepatitis C, and 1 in 100 for HIV. In general, the 'rule of 3'—30% for hepatitis B, 3% for hepatitis C and 0.3% for HIV—applies to those who are susceptible.

Table 2.8 includes diseases that may be acquired as a result of contact with blood, by accidental inoculation, skin contact or tattooing (Astbury and Baxter, 1990; Hunt, 1995).

The blood products industry, which involves the fractionation of blood to prepare therapeutic substances such as coagulation and anticoagulation factors, cytokines, interferons, antibodies and antigens may also offer some risk to workers of acquiring a hepatitis virus or HIV. The risk here is very low, but is not zero. See also Healthcare premises, below.

Table 2.8   *Bloodborne pathogens, known to have been transmitted by needlestick injuries, contact, transfusion or tattooing*

Agent	Disease
Borrelia spp	Relapsing fever
Brucella spp.	Undulant fever
Cytomegalovirus	ENT and eye infections
Haemorrhagic fever viruses	Lassa, Marburg, Ebola, Congo-Crimea fevers
Hepatitis B and C viruses	Hepatitis
Human immunodeficiency virus	AIDS
Leishmania spp.	Kala-azar
Mycobacterium leprae	Leprosy
Parvovirus B19	Arthropathy
Plasmodium malariae	Malaria
Rickettsia rickettsi	Rocky Mountain spotted fever
Treponema pallidum	Syphilis
Trypanosoma brucei gambiense	Sleeping sickness
Trypanosoma cruzi	Chagas' disease

References to these may be found in Collins (1993) and Hunt (1995).

Buildings

Fungi attack the wood, and even the plaster and brickwork, of older buildings. Disturbance, during demolition, refurbishment or redecoration, releases spores into the air. Some of these spores are allergenic, some have a carcinogenic potential (e.g. some *Aspergillus* spp.), and others are toxigenic. Damp conditions favour the growth of many of these fungi.

Allergenic bacteria, sometimes present in buildings, include *Bacillus subtilis*, the spores of which may be released during refurbishment. Johnson *et al.* (1980) reported cases of hypersensitivity pneumonia in such an instance. This organism also grows on decaying wood (Dancer, 1991), as do the actinomycetes *Faenia rectivirgula* (*Micropolyspora faenii*) and *Thermoactinomyces vulgaris* (Flannigan *et al.*, 1991) and the dry rot fungus, *Serpula lacrimans* (*Merulia lacrymans*). The use of untreated cow hair in the plastering trades carries the risk of exposure to anthrax spores (HSE, 1979).

Some of these organisms and their endotoxins have also been incriminated in humidifier fever (Rylander *et al.* 1978; Rylander and Haglind, 1984; Waldron, 1990) and in 'organic dust syndrome' (Waldron, 1990).

Aspergilli appear to be a hazard during building works, demolition and refurbishment, both to workers and to hospital patients in the vicinity of the operations (Krasinski *et al.*, 1985; Perraud *et al.*, 1987; Goodley *et al.*, 1993; Hunter, 1994) as well as to workers in road construction (Lentino *et al.*, 1982). Hay *et al.* (1995) have reviewed this problem in relation to aspergillosis in hospitals.

See also Sick building syndrome.

Cadavers (human)

Cadavers may be infected with a variety of pathogens. Mortuaries, post-mortem rooms, and funeral parlours, where bodies are embalmed or otherwise prepared for burial are therefore reservoirs of infection (McDonald, 1989; Nwanyanwu, 1989; Beck-Sague *et al.*, 1991; Healing *et al.*, 1995). The major risks at present, especially where the infection has not been diagnosed or reported to those who handle the bodies, appear to be from hepatitis B and C, HIV, tuberculosis (pulmonary and skin), enteric pathogens, staphylococcal and other skin infections; also scabies and lice. See also Blood.

Old interments

Bodies buried in old churchyards, plague pits and bones stored in charnel houses may have to be removed (the Home Office and the Environmental

Health Department must be involved). Plague bacilli, cholera and other enteric pathogens are unlikely to have survived, and the risks from anthrax and smallpox are remote (Healing *et al.*, 1995).

Eye-wash stations

Eye-wash stations in industrial premises often use water that has been in the same containers for long periods. Such stagnant water supports the growth of *Pseudomonas* species, and also of *Acanthamoeba* and *Hartmanella* species (Tyndall, 1987; Brandt *et al.* 1989; Bier and Sawyer, 1990). These organisms are common causes of corneal infections. The hazard is largely controlled by the use of disposable, sealed bottles of sterile eye-wash solutions.

Foodstuffs

Certain foodstuffs, e.g. meat, may be reservoirs of micro-organisms responsible for zoonoses. These, and products derived from milk, may contain various micro-organisms associated with food poisoning and foodborne disease. Infections with these organisms may occur during occupational activities, e.g. in handling and preparation, as well as the result of consumption (tasting!). Foodstuffs that have been associated with food poisoning, and some of the pathogens they may contain, are listed in Table 2.9.

Some of the organisms used in food manufacture may also be responsible for occupational diseases. For example, a variety of fungi, especially *Penicillium*

Table 2.9   *Food-poisoning agents and associated foods*

Organisms	Foods
Bacillus cereus	Reheated rice, soups, milk products
Campylobacter jejuni	Milk, water, poultry
Clostridium perfringens	Reheated meats
C. botulinum	Home canned or bottled vegetables, meat, fish
Listeria spp.	Cheese, dairy products, chocolate
Salmonella spp.	Poultry, eggs, meat
Staphylococcus aureus	Cold meats, dairy products
Vibrio parahaemolyticus	Seafoods
Viruses	Raw shellfish, salads washed with contaminated water

From Collins *et al.* (1995).

species, are used in cheese manufacture for ripening and flavouring. During handling and preparation for sale (i.e. washing) some of them release spores that may be allergenic.

Dried foodstuffs such as fruits and pulses may become mouldy during storage and release spores associated with lung diseases when disturbed (Crook *et al.*, 1988).

Grain dusts

Grain dusts are produced during the harvesting, drying, storage and subsequent handling of cereals (wheat, oats, barley, maize, etc.) (Lacey, 1980; HSE, 1993a,b; Pickering and Newman Taylor, 1994). The dust contains bacteria, fungal spores, insects and their parts (and also pest residues). 'Harvest dust' contains the spores of plant pathogens and saprophytic fungi. 'Stored dust', as a result of changes in humidity and temperature, contains *Aspergillus* spp. and thermophilic actinomycetes. Exposure to either may result in allergic eye and nasal reactions, occupational asthma, extrinsic allergic alveolitis (farmer's lung), 'grain fever' and chronic bronchitis. For grain dust the HSE (1993b) gives a maximum exposure limit (MEL) of 10 mg/m^3 for an 8-hour time-weighted reference period, with an indication that respiratory sensitization can result from exposure. An MEL is set on the basis that an effect threshold cannot easily be determined, and therefore the standard set takes into account the cost and practicability of available control measures.

Dust from animal feeds may also contain allergens (Pratt and May, 1984). See also Organic dusts and Plants, etc., below.

Healthcare premises; hospitals

Patients in hospitals may be infected with a variety of micro-organisms, either before admission or as a result of nosocomial transmission. Cross infection of staff, however, is comparatively rare. Tuberculosis has always been a problem, however (Patterson *et al.*, 1985; British Thoracic Society, 1990), and hospitals are reservoirs of hepatitis B: Patterson *et al.* (1985) reported that approximately 1% of health workers gave positive results in tests for the surface antigen, four times that of a comparable, non-medical, group. Hepatitis B is transmitted by sexual intercourse, from mother to child in the perinatal period and parenterally by contact with infected blood, as by drug abusers who share hypodermic syringes and needles, and occupationally from needlestick injuries. Hepatitis C is an emerging problem (Alter, 1993) and can also be occupationally acquired following needlestick injuries. The HIV virus may also be transmitted in this way (see Blood) or by contact with body fluids other than blood (see Heptonstall *et al.*, 1993). Some concern has also been expressed about the transmission of cytomegalovirus in healthcare activities (Brady, 1986).

Infectious agents to which healthcare workers are exposed are listed in Table 2.10. Apart from these, about 20 other infections are known to have resulted from needlestick injuries (Collins and Kennedy, 1988). These are listed in Table 2.11. See also Jeffries (1995) on viral agents in health care.

Occupational hazards in hospitals, including infections, have been reviewed by Gestal (1987).

Humans

Although humans may transmit many of their diseases to one another, few such diseases may be said to be occupational hazards. Some may occur from sport or recreational activities. That some diseases of occupations are prescribed (see Chapter 1) may lead us to describe them as 'occupation-mediated', e.g. as when an occupational exposure resulted in lung damage, rendering the individual more susceptible to infection from other people.

See also Cadavers (above).

Table 2.10   *Pathogens that are an occupational hazard to healthcare workers*

Bordetella spp.	Influenza viruses
Campylobacter spp.	Measles virus
Chlamydia psittaci	*Mycobacterium tuberculosis*
Corynebacterium diphtheriae	*Mycoplasma* spp.
Coxiella burnetii	Mumps virus
Creutzfeld–Jacob agent*	*Neisseria meningitidis*
Cryptosporidium spp.	Poliovirus
Cytomegalovirus	Respiratory syncytial virus
Haemorrhagic fever viruses	Rotaviruses
Helicobacter pylori	Rubella virus
Hepatitis B virus	*Salmonella* spp.
Hepatitis C virus	*Shigella* spp.
Herpes simplex virus	Varicella zoster virus
Human immunodeficiency virus	

* Uncertain.

Table 2.11 *Infections arising from needlestick injuries*

Blastomycosis	Mycobacteriosis
Brucellosis	Mycoplasmosis
Cryptococcosis	Rocky Mountain spotted fever
Diphtheria (cutaneous)	Scrub typhus
Ebola fever	Sporotrichosis
Gonorrhoea (cutaneous)	*Staphylococcus aureus* infection
Herpes	*Streptococcus pyogenes* infection
Human immunodeficiency virus infection	Syphilis
Leptospirosis	Toxoplasmosis
Malaria	Tuberculosis

Data from Collins and Kennedy (1988).

Humidifiers

See Air-conditioning plant and humidifiers.

Industrial raw and process materials

The raw materials of industries may contain large numbers of micro-organisms. These may be dispersed during handling, e.g. in 'organic dusts' (see below) or workers may come into direct contact with them. Some of them may be pathogens, although such organisms usually occur in small numbers, less than an infective dose. Opportunistic pathogens (i.e. micro-organisms that are not adapted to a parasitic existence but which may, under certain conditions, cause disease), and also those responsible for allergic reactions may be present in much larger numbers. Examples of such raw materials are (a) certain foodstuffs, e.g. poultry and seafood, intended for further processing and packaging, which may be contaminated with salmonellas, and (b) bagasse, which is sugar-cane residue after expression of the syrup and which is used to make packing and building materials. See also Foodstuffs.

Metal-working fluids—oil mists

Metal-working fluids (MWFs), also known as 'cutting oils', 'coolants', 'suds' or 'soups' are of three major types: neat oils, emulsifiable oils, and soluble synthetic substances (Travers Glass *et al.*, 1989). They are used to lubricate and cool metal parts being shaped and cut, as in lathe operations. The fluids, which are recirculated and flooded or sprayed over the tool areas, are prone to contamination with many different micro-organisms which grow well in them, and at the temperature at which the operation is performed. Bacterial counts may be as high as 10^7/ml and *Pseudomonas* species often predominate (Allsop and Seal, 1986). Aerosols ('oil mists') are also produced by the rapidly rotating machinery. Table 2.12 lists the organisms commonly found in these MWFs. Inhalation may result in allergies, respiratory infection and endo-toxicosis (Robertson *et al.*, 1988; see also Glass, 1989; Travers Glass *et al.*, 1989; Crook, 1992; HSE, 1992a).

The long-term occupational exposure limit for mineral oil mist is 5 mg/m^3. This standard is not based on the number of micro-organisms that may be present but on the chemical properties of the ingredients in mineral oils. The occupational exposure limit for oil mists is currently being reviewed by the HSE through its Advisory Committee on Toxic Substances (ACTS) and the Working Group on the Assessment of Toxic Chemicals (WATCH).

Microbiology and biomedical laboratories

Micro-organisms are concentrated in cultures in these laboratories and laboratory workers are at risk. So far this century over 5000 cases of laboratory-acquired infections have been reported with a disturbing number

Table 2.12   *Genera of micro-organisms associated with respiratory allergy and found in metal-working fluids (cutting oils)*

Aspergillus	Moraxella
Achromobacter	Morganella
Aerobacter	Pasteurella
Alkaligenes	Penicillium
Bacillus	Proteus
Botrytis	Pseudomonas
Escherichia	Sarcina
Enterobacter	Staphylococcus
Flavobacterium	Streptococcus
Geotrichum	Serratia
Klebsiella	Torulopsis
Micrococcus	

Adapted from Crook (1991), data from Allsopp and Seal (1986) and Travers Glass *et al.* (1989) reproduced by permission of *Laboratory News*.

of deaths. The number of different agents involved exceeds 120 (Collins, 1993). Fortunately, the 'escape' of dangerous pathogens from laboratories, with resulting infections among the general public, has happened on rare occasions only. The greatest hazard from these laboratories occurs when discarded cultures are not sterilized before final disposal (Collins and Kennedy, 1993). Work with pathogens, both in laboratories and in industry, is controlled under the updated *Control of Substances Hazardous to Health Regulations 1994*. This now provides a separate schedule on special provisions relating to biological agents. Biological agents have been defined under these regulations as 'any micro-organism, cell culture or human endoparasite, including any which have been genetically modified, which may cause infection, toxicity or otherwise create a hazard to human health'.

Microscopes

Eye infections in industrial settings have been reported as a result of several people using the same microscopes. A variety of micro-organisms, including *Staphylococcus aureus*, other staphylococci, corynebacteria, *Bacillus* spp, Gram-negative bacilli, adenoviruses and other viruses and fungi, have been incriminated (Olcerst, 1987; Doyle *et al.*, 1989; Paul *et al.*, 1989). Infections from this mode of transmission have not been reported in biomedical laboratories.

Organic dusts

These dusts, which include grain dusts (see above) are generated in a number of farming and industrial processes. In factories, exposure is usually controlled by engineering methods and adequate ventilation systems. These methods are not feasible in open air workplaces, such as farms, municipal waste-handling facilities, landfill sites, etc. The dusts contain large numbers of various micro-organisms, notably Gram-negative bacilli, which release endotoxins when they die and disintegrate. The main hazard from organic dusts is respiratory allergy, manifesting as asthma, extrinsic allergic alveolitis or the organic dust syndrome (Salkinoja-Salonen *et al.*, 1982; Rylander, 1986; Waldron, 1990). Intestinal symptoms have also occurred.

Plants and plant materials

Many fungi and some bacteria are parasites or commensals of plants. Many fungi develop structures, such as conidia, aerial fruiting bodies or specialized hyphal elements, that favour air dispersal. This is assisted by wind and rain.

The agents of concern here affect cereal and crop plants, including trees and shrubs, and also sphagnum moss. Harvesting and subsequent handling disturbs these organisms and their spores then become airborne and may be dispersed over a wider area than under natural circumstances. Storage at temperatures above the ambient (up to 65°C) and with water content above 30%, encourages the growth of thermophilic fungi and actinomycetes and subsequent disturbance releases very large numbers of spores which are allergenic and possibly toxigenic (Lacey *et al.*, 1972; Lacey and Crook, 1988; Lacey, 1989a,b; Crook, 1994). See also Grain dusts and Organic dusts above. Table 2.13 includes fungi and actinomycetes that may release their spores into the air and which are of occupational significance.

Table 2.13   *Fungi and actinomyces found on plants, etc. that produce spores associated with respiratory disease*

Absidia corymbifera	*Paecilomyces farinosus*
A. ramosa	*Penicillium piceum*
Alternaria alternata	*P. miczynski*
Aphanocladium album	*P. purpurogenum*
Arthrinium phaeospermum	*P. roquefortii*
Aspergillus clavatus	*P. herquei*
A. fumigatus	*P. camembertii*
A. terreus	*Pleurotis ostreatus*
A. niger	*Puccinia gaminis*
A. umbrosus	*Serpula lacrimans*
A. flavus	*Sporobolomyces roseus*
Aureobasidium pullulans	*Thermoactinomyces vulgaris*
Cladosporium fulvum	*T. sachari*
C. herbarum	*T. thalphilus*
Cryptostroma corticale	*Tilletia caries*
Epicoccus nigrum	*Ustilago avenae*
Faenia rectivirgula	*U. hordei*
Graphium spp.	*U. nuda*
Rhizomucor pusillus	*Verticillium lecani*
Nocardia asteroides	

Some names have been changed in accordance with current nomenclature. Derived mostly from Lacey *et al.* (1972) and Lacey (1989a).

Sewage and sewage sludge

Sewage, by its nature, contains very large numbers of micro-organisms, many of which are pathogens, e.g. salmonellas, listeria, and opportunistic pathogens as well as a variety of viruses (West, 1991). These may contaminate the local environment. Aerosols, which are generated during processing, will contain large numbers of faecal and other organisms, as well as their endotoxins. Apart from leptospiras, which are added to sewage by rat urine, two agents of current interest which seem to offer a particular hazard to sewage workers are *Giardia lamblia* (Heap and McCullough, 1991) and hepatitis A virus (Shakespeare and Poole, 1993). Treated and untreated sewage and sewage sludges are also spread on land as fertilizers or soil conditioners, when agricultural workers, as well as cultivated vegetables, become exposed to their microbial content (Rylander *et al.* 1976, 1983). Timothy and Mepham (1984) reported an outbreak of infectious hepatitis among sewage sludge spreaders.

Table 2.14 lists some pathogens that are not uncommon in sewage and sewage sludge. In addition, the materials contain large numbers of Gram-negative bacilli which may release endotoxins when they disintegrate.

Soils

Soils contain large numbers of microbial species, including opportunistic pathogens. Digging and other disturbances may release some of these into the air, or they may infect injuries sustained during agricultural or horticultural activities. Apart from *Clostridium tetani* and other clostridia, *Escherichia coli*

Table 2.14   *Pathogens of occupational significance that may be present in sewage*

Campylobacter jejuni	Astroviruses
Enteropathogenic *E. coli*	Coxsackie viruses
Erysipelothrix rhusiopathiae	Enteroviruses
Leptospira interrogans	Hepatitis A virus
Listeria monocytogenes	Poliovirus
Pseudomonas spp.	*Ascaris lumbricoides*
Salmonella spp.	*Acanthamoeba* spp.
Shigella spp.	*Cryptosporidium* spp.
Staphylococcus aureus	*Giardia lamblia*
	Naegleria spp.
	Taenia spp.

0157 has been found in garden soil (Cieslak *et al.*, 1993), and *Legionella longbeachae* in potting soil in relation to two cases of legionellosis (Crawford and Grant, 1994).

Wastes

Industrial wastes

The wastes and effluents from industries may contain a variety of organisms used in processing, and others that have multiplied in the waste afterwards. Fluid effluents may be discharged, deliberately or accidentally, into water courses (Brown *et al.*, 1987; Winkler and Park, 1992). Building wastes may be contaminated with bacteria and fungi whose spores are associated with allergies (see Buildings, above).

Municipal solid waste

This is the official title for domestic or household waste. It is a good culture medium and contains very large numbers of a variety of micro-organisms, up to 6.8×10^8 per gram. Some of these release large amounts of endotoxins when they die. Organisms and endotoxins are released into the atmosphere during collection, compaction, especially at waste transfer stations, and when tipped on landfill sites (Crook *et al.* 1987; Collins and Kennedy, 1992, 1993). The microbial content of municipal solid waste is shown in Table 2.15.

Table 2.15   *Genera of micro-organisms found in household and clinical waste*

*Acinetobacter**	*Listeria*†
*Alkaligenes**	*Micrococcus*
Bacillus	*Proteus*
Bacteroides	*Pseudomonas**
*Citrobacter**	*Staphylococcus*
Clostridium	*Streptococcus pyogenes**
*Enterobacter**	*Serratia**
Enterococcus	Yeasts
*Escherichia**	Mould fungi
*Klebsiella**	

* Potential endotoxin producers.
† Not found in clinical waste.
Data mainly from Crook *et al.* (1987) and Collins and Kennedy (1993).

Clinical waste

This is waste generated as a result of clinical investigative procedures and medical and surgical treatment. It is likely to contain pathogenic organisms but as its collection, transport and disposal (incineration) are carefully regulated it is not an important source or reservoir of infection. When this waste is improperly handled, however, as in the careless disposal of hollow or solid needles, needlestick injuries with subsequent infection can occur (Collins and Kennedy, 1993).

Table 2.15 includes the micro-organisms that are commonly found in clinical waste (excluding microbiology laboratory waste). The collection and disposal of clinical waste is now regulated. For details see HSE (1993e) and London Waste Regulation Authority (1994).

Water

Natural waters, streams, rivers and lakes usually have high microbial counts. The numbers are augmented from the faeces and urine of animals and are greatly increased when human sewage is added, when the flora will also include pathogenic bacteria, viruses, protozoa and helminths (Tyler, 1985; West and Locke, 1990; West, 1991). These waters, and seawater similarly polluted by sewage, constitute major reservoirs of infections. Water may become aerosolized and contribute to air pollution.

Rivers and streams may be contaminated with industrial wastes that either contain process organisms (Winkler and Park, 1992) or nutrients that allow other organisms, normally present in low numbers, to flourish and multiply.

Currently, cryptosporidiosis has assumed some importance because of the presence of the organisms in some drinking waters (Casemore, 1990; (UK) Departments of Environment and Health, 1990).

Opportunistic mycobacteria, *Mycobacterium kansasii*, *M. avium-intracellulare* and *M. xenopi*, are often present in natural and piped waters (Collins *et al.*, 1984) and may be inhaled in aerosols.

Recreational spas and whirlpools offer a suitable environment for the proliferation of *Pseudomonas* species which may cause skin conditions, and *Aeromonas hydrophila*, associated with gastrointestinal and pulmonary infections in swimmers. *Naegleria fowleri*, which, if inhaled, may cause meningitis, *Mycobacterium marinum*, responsible for swimming pool granuloma and *Legionella* species may also be present in these pools. A nosocomial outbreak of legionellosis has been associated with the inhalation of shower mists (Anon., 1988) and with aerosols from a jacuzzi (Goldberg *et al.*, 1989). Blue-green algae (Cyanophyta) may proliferate in warm weather, forming

Table 2.16   *Waterborne diseases*

Cholera*	Hepatitis A and C
Typhoid fever	Giardiasis
Paratyphoid fever	Cryptosporidiosis
Shigellosis	Amoebic dysentery*
Leptospirosis	Schistosomiasis*
Legionellosis	Acanthamoebiasis
Naegleria meningitis	Blue-green algae toxicosis

* Not in the UK.

'blooms'. These may produce toxins which may give rise to health problems if there is skin contact or ingestion (Hunter, 1991).

Table 2.16 lists waterborne infections.

3 Portals of entry and host-invader interactions

When micro-organisms or their products enter the human body they may stimulate an 'immune response'—a host-invader interaction.

Portals of entry

Micro-organisms may enter the human body through all of its orifices (although in the context of this book these include only the nose and mouth by, respectively, inhalation and ingestion), through the broken and apparently unbroken skin, and through the conjunctivae. Entry through any of these may result in infection or hypersensitivity.

Inhalation

Micro-organisms suspended in air, as dry particles, droplet nuclei or in aerosols (Chapter 2), are regularly inhaled. Although the respiratory tract is provided with mechanisms that trap many such inhaled foreign bodies, some, depending on their size, may reach the bronchi, bronchioli or even the alveoli.

Pathogenic bacteria and viruses are the most likely particles to escape the protective mechanisms and reach the lower parts of the respiratory tract, where they may initiate infections. Pathogenic micro-organisms, however, are often selective in the sites they infect or colonize. Fungal spores are frequent agents of hypersensitivity rather than infection and their entrapment and removal will depend on their size, as many of them are much larger than bacteria. Most of the spores which are 10 μm or larger in diameter will lodge in the nose, where they may initiate rhinitis. Those between 4 and 10 μm in diameter may reach the bronchi and bronchioli, where they may be responsible for asthma. But the smallest, 2–3 μm, may, like bacteria, reach the alveoli, where, instead of causing an infection, they may initiate alveolitis.

Ingestion

Many micro-organisms are ingested in food, or transferred to the mouth by contaminated fingers or objects such as cigarettes, pipes and pencils. While most such organisms are harmless or are destroyed by the gastric juices, some pathogens may reach the small intestine, where they may be responsible for a variety of intestinal infections.

Through the skin

This may be by contact or penetrating wound.

Contact

Open wounds are an obvious invitation to micro-organisms but 'entry through the unbroken skin' is often cited as a route of infection. In fact the skin is rarely unbroken, even if it appears to be intact. Microscopy will reveal large numbers of minor cuts and abrasions, many of which offer a portal for micro-organisms. Some abrasions may occur, and become infected, during work and sport. The so-called 'grass burns' are an example of the latter, as are abrasions caused by firm contact with another player's unshaven face, as in rugby scrums.

Penetrating wounds

Piercing the skin with sharp objects may inoculate the underlying tissues with micro-organisms, either from the contaminated object itself or carried in from the skin surface. Garden forks and agricultural equipment are frequently implicated. Accidental stabs with hypodermic needles (needlestick injuries) and other 'sharps' injuries are well-known sources of infections among healthcare and laboratory staff (see Table 2.8).

Through the conjunctivae

The very thin membrane of the conjunctiva is easily penetrated by micro-organisms, even in the absence of trauma. People touch and rub their eyes many more times than they suspect or admit and may easily introduce micro-organisms from the environment (Flewett, 1980).

Pathogenicity and virulence

Micro-organisms may, in general, be assigned to one of four groups: pathogens, opportunistic pathogens, commensals and saprophytes. In addition, some saprophytes are allergenic and others are toxigenic.

Pathogens are largely adapted to a parasitic existence. Some, termed obligate pathogens, are unable to survive or reproduce outside the bodies of their hosts; examples are viruses and the gonococcus, *Neisseria gonorrhoeae.* Others, e.g. the typhoid bacillus, *Salmonella typhi,* may be able to survive and reproduce in the environment but this is not their natural habitat.

Opportunistic pathogens are commensals or saprophytes that do not normally initiate disease unless they enter a host with a defective immunity or gain access by an unusual portal. Examples include *Pneumocystis carinii, Cryptosporidium* and *Mycobacterium marinum.*

Commensals are adapted to co-existence with their host without causing any harm; some are even beneficial. Examples are skin micrococci and the numerous bacterial species that inhabit the colon. They may, however, cause disease if they gain access to other parts of the body, e.g. when coliform bacilli cause urinary tract infections.

Saprophytes live in the inanimate environment and derive their nutrients from dead organic, or inorganic, matter. They contribute to soil economy and fertility by decomposing their substrates to chemicals that are assimilable by other life forms. Examples include the nitrifying bacteria.

Allergenic micro-organisms or their products provoke an adverse reaction (allergy or hypersensitivity) in the human body. Examples include the spores of certain fungi and actinomycetes.

Toxigenic micro-organisms produce highly poisonous substances termed toxins. Some pathogens, e.g. the diphtheria bacillus, *Corynebacterium diphtheriae,* and the tetanus bacilli, *Clostridium tetani,* largely owe their virulence to toxins but some saprophytes may produce enough toxins to render food or drink poisonous. Examples include the mycotoxins produced by fungi, notably *Aspergillus* species, and the toxins produced by some species of blue-green algae (*Cyanophyta*).

Pathogenicity

The ability of an organism to cause disease depends on its intrinsic virulence and the level of resistance of the host.

Virulence

Micro-organisms have evolved many determinants of virulence. Examples include mechanisms for attaching to, and entering, tissues and, in some cases, cells; the possession of capsules which prevent them from being engulfed by phagocytic cells, mechanisms to survive within phagocytic cells, and the production of toxins. There are two broad groups of toxins: *exotoxins*, which are polypeptides secreted by living bacteria; and *endotoxins* which are lipopolysaccharides in the outer layers of the cell walls of Gram-negative bacteria and which are released when dead organisms disintegrate.

Host defences and the immune system

The normal human body has a number of defences against the intrusion of micro-organisms, and mechanisms for destroying them should they gain access. These defences are non-specific, or innate, and specific.

In the first group there is the intact skin, which is an efficient barrier; there is also an antibacterial substance, lysozyme, in the saliva and the tears, and acid and enzymes in the digestive tract. Ciliated epithelium (the 'ciliary escalator') in the nasopharynx sweeps inhaled particles upwards so they may be ejected at the mouth and nose, or swallowed.

The specific human immune system has evolved to cope with a vast range of pathogenic micro-organisms and other harmful substances. The three key features of this system are recognition, response and reaction.

Recognition

The immune system distinguishes 'foreign' from 'self'. For this purpose, there is a huge diversity of lymphocytes, each capable of recognizing just one of thousands of antigenic determinants or epitopes. It was previously thought that lymphocytes recognizing 'self' epitopes were eliminated during fetal development but it is now known that they survive but are under close regulatory control. Sometimes this regulation fails and these cells are then able to react against 'self' epitopes, thereby causing various autoimmune diseases, of which rheumatoid arthritis is the best known example.

Response

Foreign antigen is taken up by a class of cells known as antigen-presenting cells (APCs) and thereby delivered to the antigen-specific lymphocytes. The APCs activate these lymphocytes so that they undergo division to form a clone of identical cells. Because of the huge diversity of antigens, the number of lymphocytes responding to one epitope is small. Clonal expansion is therefore essential for the generation of enough lymphocytes to facilitate an immune reaction.

There are several types of lymphocytes with quite different functions. The B cells are responsible for antibody synthesis and the T cells are involved in initiating and helping immune responses, especially the cell-mediated immune reactions. T cells can also be cytotoxic in that they are capable of destroying virus-infected host cells. T cells with different functions are recognizable by cell surface markers called CD (cluster differentiating) antigens. Most helper/inducer T cells are CD4+ while suppressor/cytotoxic cells are mostly CD8+.

Reaction

The activated and clonally expanded lymphocytes secrete various chemical messengers or cytokines which facilitate the actual reaction against the invading pathogen or allergen. These reactions involve antibody, complement (a group of serum proteins which, as the name suggests, assists the action of antibody), phagocytic cells of which there are two main classes, the neutrophils and the macrophages, and cytotoxic cells. Neutrophils are members of a class of white cells called granulocytes, characterized by cytoplasmic granules. The name neutrophil alludes to their neutral staining granules. Other granulocytes, termed eosinophils and basophils according to their staining properties, are involved in Type I (allergic) hypersensitivity reactions (see below).

Antibody is able to neutralize toxins, such as the diphtheria and tetanus toxins, and small viruses. It also adheres to bacteria, fungi and the larger viruses enabling them to be engulfed and destroyed by the phagocytic cells. There are five classes of human antibody, or immunoglobulin: IgG, IgM, IgA, IgD and IgE. The first two are found principally in serum and tissue fluids while IgA is also secreted into the lumen of the respiratory and alimentary tracts. IgE is involved in Type I hypersensitivity reactions (see below). No specific function has been ascribed to IgD. The enhancement of phagocytosis by antibody is termed opsonization and is aided by complement which binds to, and is activated by, antigen-antibody complexes containing IgG or IgM. Another function of complement is to attach itself to antibody-coated pathogens and to lyse their cell membranes. Excess complement activation may damage nearby 'innocent cells'. Such bystander lysis is responsible for tissue damage in Type III hypersensitivity reactions (see below).

The polymorphonuclear leucocytes are short-lived cells liberated from the bone marrow in response to acute infections. Macrophages are much longer-lived cells which, for maximum effectiveness, must be activated by T cell-derived cytokines, principally gamma interferon. They play a major role in immunity to chronic infections such as tuberculosis and many fungal diseases in which they surround the pathogens in characteristic compact aggregates termed granulomas.

Cytotoxic cells detect and destroy cells containing pathogens such as viruses, thereby exposing them to antibody and phagocytic cells. The importance of these cells in chronic bacterial diseases such as tuberculosis has recently been recognized.

Hypersensitivity reactions

These are excessive and inappropriate immune reactions to foreign antigen and cause discomfort or harm to the host. There are four main types of allergy but only two of them are of interest in the context of this book.

Type I reactions

Also called allergic, atopic or anaphylactic reactions, these are the result of antigen binding to antibody, mostly in the IgE class, on the surface of basophils and mast cells. This triggers an explosive release of histamine and other substances that cause conditions such as hay fever, asthma and urticaria.

Type III reactions

'Arthus type' reactions occur when an individual with high levels of specific antibody is exposed to the corresponding antigen. This results in the formation of immune complexes which induce tissue damage. Such reactions are usually the result of repeated occupational exposure to the antigen (usually by inhalation). Farmer's lung is an example.

4 People at risk

It is not possible to make a list of all the occupations, sports and recreational activities that offer the risk of infection or microbial allergy. Nor is it reasonable to separate 'work' from 'pleasure' as most sports and recreational activities require the services of full-time or part-time employees. Some people are more at risk than others because their normal defences are impaired, e.g. by skin diseases, pregnancy or treatment with steroids.

New occupations and activities develop and unexpected diseases may occur from time to time. Moreover, the same kinds of occupation, with the same or similar risks, may be given different names by different workers in, perhaps, different areas. The following list therefore includes several duplications of conditions.

Ambulance and paramedical staff

Exposure to blood which may be infected with hepatitis B, hepatitis C, HIV and other agents is the most serious microbiological hazard for these people.

Anatomical pathology technicians

See Mortuary and postmortem room staff.

Anglers

Both sea and freshwater anglers are exposed to waterborne infections, but unlike other watersports people they are unlikely to ingest the water. Nevertheless, there are diseases of fish which may be transferred to the hands and exposed parts of the body. These include mycobacteriosis (*Mycobacterium marinum* infection), erysipeloid (saltwater fish) and, unusually among anglers, leptospirosis. They are also at risk from cryptosporidiosis and eye infections caused by *Acanthamoeba* species (see Table 2.12).

Animal breeders and handlers

Animal breeders and handlers are exposed to the zoonotic infections of their charges. (See Tables 2.2, 2.3 and 2.4.) These workers may also develop respiratory allergies as a result of exposure to urine, dander and other animal proteins.

People who keep cats and dogs as pets and those who breed and/or board them are exposed to the zoonoses of these animals, especially toxocariasis (dogs) and toxoplasmosis (cats). Dogs may be infected with leptospires and tapeworms but fortunately hydatid disease, caused by *Echinococcus granulosus*, is rare in developed countries. Both cats and dogs are frequently infected with ringworm fungi, transmissible to humans, and with salmonellas. Cat-scratch fever is not uncommon, nor are infections with *Pasteurella multocida*.

See also Bird fanciers, Fish fanciers.

Athletes

Athletes engaged in various sports may receive injuries while in contact with soil and are therefore exposed to infections with *Clostridium* species and to sepsis.

In changing rooms and showers they may acquire fungal infections of the feet ('athlete's foot'), other ringworms and verrucas. Communal towels may also spread these agents. See also Ball-team and contact sports; Water sports; Sharp (1993, 1994).

Bagasse workers

Bagasse is obtained from the crushed stems and other parts of the sugar-cane plant after removal of the syrup. Formerly burned, it is now imported and used in the manufacture of hardboards, building board and packaging materials. Micro-organisms multiply in the raw material and large numbers of spores of several species of bacteria and fungi are produced during shipping and storage and are released when the material is disturbed (Lacey, 1971). Inhalation of these may result in a form of extrinsic allergic alveolitis termed bagassosis.

Ball-team and contact sportspeople

In sports such as rugby football and soccer the skin of players may be abraded, e.g. by beard stubble, during violent personal contact. It is then liable to infection with a number of micro-organisms. One such condition is known as 'scrumpox' or 'Herpes gladiatorum', and is of bacterial or fungal aetiology (Sharp and Adams, 1990; Sharp, 1994). Wounds, contaminated with soil, may become septic or even be infected with *Clostridium* species. Other bacterial and fungal infections (such as athlete's foot) may be acquired during exposure in communal baths and from the floors of changing rooms. Impetigo, verrucas, erysipelas, glandular fever and giardiasis may also be passed around under these conditions (Sharp, 1993, 1994).

Biotechnology and pharmaceutical industry workers

A wide variety of bacteria and fungi are used in traditional and re-combinant biotechnology (Tables 2.6 and 2.7). Although these are mostly in Group 1 of the classification of micro-organisms on the basis of hazard (Chapter 10) and therefore unlikely to cause infections, some produce spores and metabolic products, e.g. the enzyme alcalase, derived from *Bacillus* species and used in biological detergents. Inhalation of this enzyme during the production processes has resulted in asthma and other respiratory symptoms.

Other biotechnology industries that employ potentially allergenic micro-organisms are protein production (*Candida tropicalis, Methylophilus methylotrophus, Methylomonas methylonica*) and citric acid production (*Aspergillus, Penicillium* species).

Some pathogenic micro-organisms are used to manufacture vaccines and diagnostic materials. Most are in Hazard Group 2 (see Chapter 10) and have a low potential for causing infections among those who work with them. Some Hazard Group 3 organisms, however, are used in vaccine manufacture. Respiratory allergies may result from exposure to the spores of some fungi that are used in the manufacture of antibiotics.

Apart from these pathogens, contaminants may be present, e.g. in cell and tissue cultures used for propagation. Some of these, e.g. mycoplasmas and various viruses, may be hazardous to health (Beale, 1992).

Bird fanciers

This wide group includes pigeon fanciers and those who convey homing pigeons, keepers of exotic birds in aviaries, as well as pet-shop and zoo staff, and those engaged in falconry and hawking. These people are exposed to, and may inhale, the dust from feathers and droppings, resulting in a form of extrinsic allergic alveolitis termed 'bird fancier's lung' or 'bird breeder's lung'.

The dust may also contain a variety of fungal spores, the inhalation of which may result in respiratory allergies. Birds may be infected with the agent of psittacosis/ornithosis (avian chlamydiosis), as well as with salmonellas.

Building trades

See Construction workers.

Canteen staff

See Food handlers, meat trades workers.

Care staff and teachers

Young children are frequently infested with pinworms, also known as threadworms (*Enterobius vermicularis*). Child carers and nursery nurses may acquire these helminths by the hand-to-mouth route from the faeces, perianal areas and soiled clothing of their charges. These carers are also exposed to cytomegalovirus, excreted in faeces and saliva and not infrequently found in (symptomless) young children. Bacterial dysentery (mostly the Sonne type) and enterotoxigenic *Escherichia coli* enteritis are also occupational hazards of child carers and nursery nurses.

Those who care for the incontinent are also exposed to hepatitis A virus, excreted in faeces.

Cereal and grain handlers

These commodities are naturally infected with a variety of fungi and actinomycetes (see Farmers and farmworkers). Spores may be released in large numbers during harvesting, when the grain is disturbed in silos and during transport. Inhalation may result in respiratory symptoms, although asthma in grain handlers is usually attributable to the inhalation of grain dust rather than micro-organisms. Malt worker's lung is due to the inhalation of *Aspergillus clavatus*, present as a contaminant in barley which is used in the production of whisky.

Chiropodists

Although exposure to ringworm fungi (in particular *Trichophyton rubrum*) is a common hazard to chiropodists, there is also the risk of exposure to bloodborne diseases if the patient is inadvertently cut and there is contact with blood.

Construction workers

The demolition or refurbishment of old buildings frequently results in the release of large numbers of fungal and bacterial spores associated with respiratory allergies. Imported cow hair that has escaped disinfection may contain anthrax spores. Roofers may be exposed to pigeon faeces which contain *Chlamydia psittaci*, the agent of ornithosis (Woodhead, 1994). Excavating and earth moving carries the risk of exposure to the spores of tetanus bacilli.

Contact sportspeople

See Ball-team sportspeople.

Cooks

See Food handlers, meat trades workers.

Country walkers

Country walkers and ramblers may be exposed, in some areas, to the ticks that harbour the agent of Lyme disease, *Borrelia burgdorferi*. They may also be pricked by the spines of plants and develop sporotrichosis if the plants are carrying the fungus *Sporotrichum* (*Sporothrix*) *schenckii*. Injuries contaminated with soil may result in tetanus.

Custodial staff

Prison officers and others who are responsible for custodial care may be victims of aggression and, therefore, exposed to bloodborne diseases. They may also be exposed to tubercle bacilli, e.g. from undiagnosed people who are on remand.

Cyclists

Cyclists, especially those who engage in cross-country and 'mountain' cycling may be exposed to the agents of Lyme disease and sporotrichosis. Injuries contaminated with soil may result in tetanus or mycobacteriosis.

Dentists and dental assistants

Like other healthcare workers, dentists and their assistants may be exposed to bloodborne infections (hepatitis B and C, and HIV). Recently, concern has been expressed about *Helicobacter pylori*, associated with gastric ulcers, and present in dental tartar, which may be dispersed in aerosols during drilling and scaling (Malaty *et al.*, 1992). The risk of exposure to other agents in aerosols generated by high speed drills is under consideration (see Lewis and Boe, 1992; Carter, 1992).

Divers

See Water industry workers and sportspeople.

Dock workers

Leptospirosis is not uncommon among dock workers who are in regular contact with water which may be contaminated with rat urine and faeces. They may also be exposed to anthrax spores in imported hairs and hides. Eye infections, caused, e.g. by *Acanthamoeba* species and adenoviruses ('shipyard eye', Anon., 1981), also occur. These workers are also subject to respiratory allergies as a result of inhaling organic dusts, released during the handling of cargoes.

Ear piercers

Ear piercers are exposed to bloodborne infections, e.g hepatitis B and C and HIV. They are also exposed to ringworm fungi as a result of close contact with hair of their clients.

Environmental health inspectors

These local government officers include meat and food inspections among their activities (see Meat trade workers, Food handlers). They are also exposed to a variety of infectious diseases during their investigations in cases of communicable diseases, and also to various agents of respiratory allergies during the inspection of dilapidated premises.

Equestrians and stable staff

People who are in regular contact with horses are at risk from glanders (caused by *Pseudomonas mallei*). Tetanus, if wounds are contaminated with horse faeces, is also possible. A fatal disease of horses, transmissible to humans and caused by a morbillivirus, has been reported in Australia (Murray *et al.*, 1995). Asthma and farmer's lung may result from exposure to fungal and actino-mycete spores on hay and straw.

Farmers and farm workers

This broad group includes those who are engaged in animal husbandry and dairy farming, and arable farmers who grow, harvest and pack cereals and other field crops.

Animal husbandry

Workers in this group are at risk from zoonoses, including anthrax (although this is rare), erysipeloid, *Streptococcus suis* infection (also rare), brucellosis, listeriosis, orf, ovine chlamydiosis, Q fever, leptospirosis, bovine tuberculosis, yersiniosis, salmonellosis, mycobacteriosis, milker's nodules, ringworms, aspergillosis and cryptosporidiosis. Roundworm infestations occur but tape-worm infestations are uncommon in the UK. There is also the risk of fungal allergies involving spores of fungi and actinomycetes, especially among workers who handle fodder. Piggery workers are exposed to a wide range of airborne micro-organisms, some of which are associated with respiratory disease. Pregnant women engaged in lambing are exposed to *Chlamydia psittaci* the agent of enzootic abortion of ewes (ovine chlamydiosis) (Buxton, 1986; HSE, 1993c). There is also concern about the possible hazards of exposure to the agent of 'mad cow disease' (bovine spongiform encephalitis, BSE).

Farm dairy staff who make cheese may suffer from cheese-maker's lung as a result of inhaling spores of *Aspergillus clavatus*, released when the mould is washed off the cheese before preparation for sale.

Arable farmers

Those engaged in crop production are more at risk from microbial allergies than infections. These allergies range from rhinitis, through asthma to extrinsic alveolitis. Large numbers of spores of fungi and bacteria are released during harvesting (see Table 2.13, p. 26). Post processing of hay, under certain conditions of warmth and moisture, release the spores of *Thermoactinomyces vulgaris* and *Faenia rectivirgula* (*Micropolyspora faeni*), associated with farmer's lung, grain worker's lung and mushroom worker's lung. *Klebsiella* species are often present in wood shavings and sawdust used as litter and may release endotoxins into the air when the litter is disturbed. *Mycobacterium terrae*, a soil organism, may infect wounds sustained during agricultural activities. Foliage may also harbour *Sporotricum schenckii*, which may infect minor skin lesions, giving rise to sporotrichosis. Exceptionally, this fungus may cause lung disease, resembling tuberculosis.

Agricultural workers are also exposed to silage, where tapeworms may be found as well as *Nocardia* species and *Listeria monocytogenes*. Sewage sludge, used as fertilizer, etc. may contain a variety of pathogens, including salmonellas, leptospirosis, giardia, cryptosporidia and hepatitis A virus.

Fellmongers

See hair, hide and wool workers.

Fertilizer manufacturing workers

The raw materials include bones, bonemeal, hooves and horns, all of which may contain anthrax spores.

Field sportspeople

Any activity that involves contact with soil and plant material leads to exposure to clostridial infections (e.g. tetanus) and septic infections of cuts and scratches. Also sporotrichosis, caused by contact with spiny and prickly foliage which often harbours *Sporothrix schenkii*.

First aid workers

Those who render first aid to victims of accidents run the risk of exposure to blood and therefore to bloodborne diseases, especially hepatitis B and C, and possibly HIV.

Fishermen and fishery workers

These people are particularly at risk from erysipeloid, leptospirosis and mycobacteriosis.

Fish fanciers

Fish fanciers often specialize in tropical and other exotic fish. Some of these may be infected with *Mycobacterium marinum*, which is shed into the water of the aquarium. If this organism enters the skin through minor cuts and abrasions the condition known as fish tank granuloma or fish-fancier's finger may result. The water may also contain *Pseudomonas* and *Aeromonas* species, opportunist pathogens which may be responsible for skin infections.

Florists; flower arrangers

Sporotrichosis and streptococcal infections may result from injuries caused by infected thorns, spines and prickles.

Food handlers

Cooks, canteen staff and other people who handle food, especially the raw products, may encounter salmonellas in infective doses, as well as other food poisoning agents (see Table 2.5, p. 15). Candidiasis is not unknown among food handlers, nor is trichinosis.

Forensic scientists and scene of crime officers

The principal risks in these occupations are exposure to the blood of victims of crimes, which may be infected with a hepatitis virus and possibly with HIV.

Foresters

In areas where there are deer there is the risk of Lyme disease. Foresters are also exposed to occupational asthma and extrinsic alveolitis as a result of exposure to organic (especially wood) dusts. Injuries contaminated with soil may result in clostridial infections (e.g. tetanus) or mycobacteriosis.

Funeral staff and morticians

In spite of the precautions normally taken by hospital staff in dealing with the dead, those who prepare cadavers for funerals, especially embalmers, may be exposed to blood, infected, e.g. with hepatitis B and C viruses and HIV, either by contact or sharps injuries (hollow needles). There is also the risk from enteric pathogens as a result of the leakage of faeces and of staphylococcal and other skin infections, and scabies and lice infestation (McDonald, 1989; Nwanyanwu, 1989; Beck-Sague *et al.*, 1991; Healing *et al.*, 1995). See also Blood; Cadavers (human); Mortuary and Postmortem room staff.

Game keepers

Game keepers may be exposed to the ornithosis/psittacosis agent and also to ticks that carry the Lyme disease spirochaete.

Gardeners

Gardeners and horticultural workers who suffer penetrating wounds while at work are at risk from tetanus and possibly gas gangrene bacilli. Sepsis of minor wounds is not uncommon. Rose growers seem to be at risk from sporotrichosis, as the fungus *Sporothrix schenckii* is often present on rose thorns. This fungus is known to be responsible for cases of pulmonary sporotrichosis. Enteropathogenic *Escherichia coli* (0.157) has been isolated from manured garden soil (Cieslak *et al.*, 1993) and *Legionella longbeachae* from potting compost (Crawford and Grant, 1994). Imported bonemeal fertilizer that has escaped disinfection may contain anthrax spores. *Mycobacterium terrae*, present in soil, may infect wounds sustained during gardening activities.

Glue and gelatin manufacturing workers

Bones, hooves and horns are used in this industry and may contain anthrax spores.

Groundsmen

Groundsmen are in contact with soil and are therefore at risk from tetanus if they suffer penetrating wounds in the course of their work and also from other infections to which gardeners are exposed (see Gardeners). Groundsmen in parks are also exposed to toxocaras when they mow grass fouled by dog faeces.

Hairdressers

The ringworm fungi, responsible for tinea capitis (caused by *Microsporum audouini*), and favus (caused by *Trichophyton schonleinii*) may be transmitted from clients to hairdressers.

Healthcare staff

Medical and nursing staff, as well as their assistants and hospital lay staff, are at risk from any number of infections that may be acquired from patients. Tables 2.10 and 2.11 list micro-organisms that are occupational risks for healthcare workers.

At present the main concerns are hepatitis B, hepatitis C and HIV infection. Needlestick and other 'sharps' injuries, in which very small amounts of blood may be transferred from patient to staff, may transmit a wide variety of bloodborne and other infections. These are listed in Table 2.11 (p. 23).

Hepatitis A virus may be present in the faeces of hospital patients. See also Patterson *et al.* (1985). Tuberculosis is an ever-present risk (British Thoracic Society, 1990), particularly in view of the emergence of multidrug-resistant tubercle bacilli (Sepkowitz, 1994). Of recent interest are reports of infections of pregnant women with cytomegalovirus, which may affect the fetus (Tookey and Peckham, 1991; Tookey and Logan, 1994) and of respiratory syncytial virus. The skin of healthcare workers may be colonized by methicillin-resistant *Staphylococcus aureus*. Although these organisms may not affect the worker they may be transmitted to patients who are in a poor state of health.

Jeffries (1995) has reviewed viruses that may be transmitted from patients to staff.

Hide, hair and wool workers

Traditionally, these workers, including those who work in tanneries and in brush manufacture are at risk from anthrax, as the spores of *Bacillus anthracis* not infrequently contaminate the raw materials, especially those that are imported. Dockers who handle the imports are also at risk, although this has been reduced by obligatory disinfection.

The epithets 'wool sorter's disease' for pulmonary anthrax, and 'malignant pustule' for cutaneous infection are now considered to be redundant. Occupational anthrax is relatively uncommon nowadays.

Anthrax is not the only disease that may be acquired from hides, hairs and wool fleeces; there is a potential for erysipeloid, Q fever and ringworm infections.

Horse copers

See Equestrians and stable staff.

Hunters

Hunters, especially those who hunt on foot in well-wooded areas, may encounter *Ixodes* ticks which may transmit the spirochaete of Lyme disease.

Incinerator operators

These workers may be exposed to micro-organisms in waste and refuse as well as to endotoxins. Those who handle clinical waste containers may be exposed to pathogens released from damaged containers.

Kitchen staff

See Food handlers, meat trades workers.

Knackers

Knackers, who slaughter horses, may encounter cases of glanders, from which they may acquire *Pseudomonas mallei* infection. Those who remove diseased, dead and dying farm animals are exposed to the zoonoses of those animals, including, possibly, morbillivirus infection (see Equestrians, etc. above).

Laboratory animal technicians and assistants

These workers are at risk from any of the zoonoses of their charges (see Table 2.4, p. 14).

Laundry workers

Laundry workers may handle clothing contaminated with the spores of various ringworm fungi and may therefore become infected. Prolonged exposure of the hands to water, especially that containing detergents, may predispose to skin infections. Infected clothing has been responsible for the spread of Q fever to laundry workers (Oliphant *et al.*, 1949).

Maltsters

Maltsters, in common with other people who work with cereals, may develop allergies to the spores of various fungi. The condition known as malt worker's lung is associated with *Aspergillus clavatus*, a contaminant of barley used in making whisky.

Meat inspectors

Meat inspectors are subject to the same series of zoonotic infections as meat trades workers (see also Tobie and McCullough, 1961).

Meat trades workers

Abattoir workers include lairage staff, slaughterhouse workers, butchers and meat inspectors, and also unskilled operatives who are responsible for removing offal and for general cleaning work. All are at risk from the zoonotic diseases of cattle, sheep and pigs. These include anthrax (rare), erysipeloid, *Streptococcus suis* infection (also rare), brucellosis, listeriosis, orf, Q fever, pasteurellosis, helminthiasis, leptospirosis, tuberculosis, mycobacteriosis and ringworm infections.

Medical laboratory staff

Laboratory-acquired infections have an extensive literature of their own (Collins, 1993). Almost all of the organisms encountered in clinical laboratories have been implicated at one time or other, but at present hepatitis B and bowel infections are the most frequently reported (Grist and Emslie, 1991). Infections with exotic micro-organisms occur occasionally among laboratory staff who handle specimens and cultures sent from abroad for investigation.

Medical practitioners

See Healthcare staff.

Metal workers

Lathe operators and other metal workers use metal-working fluids (cutting oils) to cool and lubricate their processes. These oil–water emulsions are not infrequently contaminated with bacteria such as *Pseudomonas* species and staphylococci, which may cause skin infections and respiratory symptoms (Crook, 1992). See Table 2.12 (p. 24).

Microbiologists

Medical microbiologists are at risk from the same infections as medical laboratory staff (see above). Non-medical microbiologists may consider that they are not at risk as they do not handle infectious or clinical material but those who examine food and other commodities may concentrate to infective doses the small numbers of pathogens, e.g. salmonellas, that not infrequently contaminate such materials.

Miners

Traditionally, miners were at risk from hookworm disease but this was the result of inadequate sanitation in mines. When faeces containing the eggs of the hookworms *Ankylostoma duodenale* and *Necator americanus* are deposited in moist, warm places the larval forms emerge and can penetrate intact human skin. Today, ankylostomiasis is encountered only in some tropical and subtropical countries.

Miners are also at risk of developing pneumoconiosis and silicosis which predispose to tuberculosis.

Mortuary and postmortem room staff

These workers, including anatomical pathology technicians, are exposed to hepatitis B and C, possibly to HIV, and also to lung and skin infections ('prosector's wart') with tubercle bacilli (especially from cases undiagnosed during life) and any other pathogens with which the cadaver was infected. Transmissible spongiform encephalopathies must also be considered. See also Funeral staff and morticians.

Mushroom growers and pickers

Mushroom grower's lung is a form of extrinsic allergic alveolitis that occurs among staff in this industry and results from exposure to the spores of *Thermoactinomyces vulgaris* and *Faenia rectivirgula* (*Micropolyspora faeni*), released when the compost is 'turned'. The spores of some mushrooms are allergenic but the fungi grown in the UK are usually picked at the button stage. The varieties grown in Europe, however, are allowed to open before picking, when their spores may be released into the air.

Nursery nurses

See Child care staff.

Nurses

See Healthcare staff.

Office workers

Respiratory and other infections that are transmitted from person to person in offices cannot be considered as occupational diseases. In some buildings, however, such as those with air conditioning, sick building syndrome (SBS) has been described (Chapter 5). This seems to occur mostly at the beginning of the week, after the air conditioning is restarted after the weekend. It consists of vague symptoms such as lethargy, tiredness, headache, and eye, nose and throat irritation. While some studies have shown a relationship between SBS and the numbers of fungal spores and hyphal fragments in the air, the cause is likely to be multifactorial. In offices, cases and outbreaks of humidifier fever (Chapter 5) and Pontiac fever (fever and chills with myalgia, malaise and headache, and caused by *Legionella pneumophila*) may occur. Legionnaire's disease often results from colonization of air-conditioning cooling towers with these organisms, which then spread in aerosols to the surrounding area.

Orienteering

See Country walking.

Park keepers

See Gardeners, Groundsmen.

Pet-shop staff

See Animal handlers, Bird fanciers, Fish fanciers.

Pharmaceutical industries

See Biotechnology.

Physicians

See Healthcare workers.

Pigeon fanciers

See Bird fanciers, Animal handlers.

Police officers

Police officers are not infrequently in contact with human blood and body fluids when they attend road and other accidents and render first aid, as well as in the immediate investigation of homicides, assaults and suicides. They are also likely to be victims of aggression. They are therefore at risk of infection with hepatitis B or C, even with HIV.

Postmortem room attendants

See Mortuary and postmortem room staff.

Poultry workers

In addition to the infections that may occur among agricultural workers and bird fanciers (e.g. ornithosis (psittacosis)), poultry workers and those who process poultry, e.g. killing, plucking and eviscerating the birds for the market may be exposed to ornithosis, to the virus of Newcastle disease, which is known to cause human disease (conjunctivitis), and also to papillomavirus infections. Erysipeloid is another hazard. Exposure to organic dusts (containing e.g. endotoxins) in poultry houses may lead to respiratory problems (Hagman, 1990). Environmental monitoring of inhalable endotoxins in poultry houses has yielded levels between 8 and 200 $\mu g/g$ of dust. An airborne concentration of 0.5 $\mu g/m^3$ has been suggested as the minimum level that produces reaction in humans (Anon., 1987).

Pregnant women

Many pregnant women often continue to work until the end of the second trimester. Rubella and cytomegalovirus infections are known to damage the fetus. There is an EC Directive (European Commission, 1992), implemented in the UK by amendments to the *Management of Health and Safety at Work Regulations 1992*, which specifically prohibits pregnant women working in occupations where they are exposed to toxoplasmas (see also Thomas and Joynson, 1994) and (unless they are immunized) rubella.

The HSE (1993c) suggests that pregnant women should not assist at lambing as the agent of enzootic abortion of ewes (ovine chlamydiosis, caused by *Chlamydia psittaci*) can pose a risk to the fetus (Buxton, 1986).

Print workers

Humidifiers of various kinds are used in the printing industries, with the consequent risk of humidifier fever (Chapter 5).

Prison officers

See Custodial staff.

Prostitutes

Apart from the usual sexually transmitted diseases such as syphilis, gonorrhoea and herpes, prostitutes are at risk from HIV, hepatitis B and C, and also from skin diseases, including scabies and infestations with lice, acquired during close personal contact with their clients.

Quarry workers

Silicosis is an industrial disease of quarry workers and those who process stony materials. This disease predisposes to tuberculosis.

Rabbit fanciers

See Animal handlers.

Ramblers

See Country walkers.

Refuse and waste workers

Although there appear to be few infectious hazards in the handling of municipal refuse, waste workers are exposed to dusts, especially at transfer stations and landfill sites. Various respiratory symptoms have been reported. In addition, allergic reactions to endotoxins, generated in large amounts, can occur as a result of the growth in the refuse of Gram-negative bacilli (*Escherichia, Enterobacter, Klebsiella, Pseudomonas* species, etc.) (see Chapter 6).

There are also health risks in the handling of clinical waste (Collins and Kennedy, 1992, 1993).

River and canal workers

The important occupational disease of these workers is leptospirosis but they are also exposed to cryptosporidiosis, giardiasis and a variety of other infections including *Acanthamoeba* eye infections and keratinophilic fungi. (See Table 2.16, p. 30.)

Seafarers

There appears to be a high incidence of tuberculosis among seamen (Oliver, 1979).

Sewage workers

Leptospirosis is the main microbial hazard of sewermen and sewage works staff, but they are also exposed to *Giardia lamblia* (Heap and McCullough, 1991) and hepatitis A (Shakespeare and Poole, 1993) as well as salmonellas, campylobacters and a variety of entero- and other viruses (Tyler, 1985; West, 1991). Inhalation of aerosols containing micro-organisms and endotoxins may result in bowel disorders and, in some cases, respiratory allergies (Rylander *et al.* 1983). HSE issues useful leaflets (Appendix 2).

Shepherds

Shepherds are as subject to zoonoses as other farm workers but they are particularly exposed to the agents of Q fever and orf. Female shepherds, if pregnant, are at risk from the agent of enzootic abortion of ewes (see Farmer's and farm workers).

Slaughterhouse workers

See Meat trades workers.

Soldiers

Military personnel are in frequent contact with soil and therefore with clostridia, which may infect penetrating wounds and cause tetanus and/or gas gangrene, although most soldiers are vaccinated and receive regular booster doses to keep up their immunity from such infections. Use of communal baths and accommodation may predispose to ringworm and other skin infections. Dysentery is a well-known problem of active service, where sanitary arrangements may be primitive or non-existent.

Soil and earth movers

Septic and clostridial infections of wounds, acquired from soil, are the main microbial hazards of these occupations.

Spa and whirlpool ('jacuzzi') users

Continued exposure of the skin to warm water carries the risk of skin infections due to (mainly) *Pseudomonas* species and staphylococci. Legionellosis has also been reported among spa bathers (Jones *et al.*, 1982), as has *Acanthamoeba* keratitis (Kilvington and White, 1994).

Stable staff

See Equestrians.

Surgeons

Surgeons appear to be particularly at risk from needlestick and other sharps injuries, followed by infection with hepatitis B or C viruses and possibly HIV. (See Healthcare staff.)

Tannery workers

See Hair, hides and wool workers.

Tattooists

Tattooists' customers may bleed and the operators are therefore at risk from hepatitis B and C, possibly HIV.

Taxidermists

Taxidermists are at risk from zoonoses; those who prepare birds are particularly at risk from psittacosis (avian chlamydiosis).

Teachers

See Care staff.

Timber workers

Certain timbers, when being prepared for sawing, release clouds of fungal or actinomycete spores, which, if inhaled, may be allergenic.

Veterinary surgeons and staff

Veterinary staff are subject to most zoonoses (see Animal breeders and handlers, Farmers, animal husbandry, and Tables 2.2, 2.3 and 2.4, pp. 12, 13 and 14).

Water industry workers and watersports people

Water workers include professional divers and river and canal workers (see above). Water sports include canoeing, sailing, skin diving, swimming and various other 'aquasports'. While leptospirosis is the main concern for workers and sportspeople, contact with and ingestion of natural waters, fresh or sea, that are often contaminated with sewage may lead to gastrointestinal infections, e.g. salmonellosis, helminthiasis, cryptosporidiosis, giardiasis, and to disease caused by viruses, e.g. enterovirus, astrovirus, calicivirus, hepatitis A and to Norwalk viruses (West, 1991).

Skin infections such as mycobacteriosis (infection with *Mycobacterium marinum*) can occur. Some waters and their sediments contain keratinophilic fungi. Eye infections, both pyogenic and associated with *Acanthamoeba*, also occur. Ear infections are not uncommon. Prolonged exposure to water may soften the skin and predispose to skin infections.

Wild animal handlers

See Animal breeders and handlers. Tables 2.2, 2.3, 2.4 and 2.5 list some relevant zoonoses.

Zoo keepers

See Animal breeders and handlers. Tables 2.2, 2.3, 2.4 and 2.5 list some relevant zoonoses.

5 Infections

Some of the infections described here are prescribed, others are notifiable under the *Public Health (Infectious Diseases) Regulations 1988* (see Tables 1.1 and 1.5, pp. 3 and 8). Several are neither, but all are reportable under RIDDOR.

Ankylostomiasis (ancylostomiasis)

This is a prescribed disease (Category B4) although it is very rare in the UK. The causative organisms are hookworms: *Ankylostoma duodenale* in Europe and *Necator americana* in the USA and other parts of the world. Rarer species are *A. braziliensis, A. caninum* and *A. ceylanicum*. These helminths do not require alternative hosts. The eggs are passed in the faeces and, given a high ambient temperature and humidity, hatch into larvae that penetrate the skin, usually through abrasions on the feet, where they may cause localized macules called 'ground itch'. The larvae then migrate via the lymphatics and blood to the lungs and intestine, where they produce more eggs.

A group of people at risk in temperate climes are miners who work under insanitary conditions. Prescription of ankylostomiasis in the UK is 'work in or about a mine'.

In the USA, South America, India and South East Asia the hookworms of cats and dogs (*A. braziliensis*) may penetrate the skin and migrate locally, causing a creeping eruption known as *larva migrans*. Larvae reaching the lung may cause Loeffler's syndrome, a condition also caused by *Ascaris lumbricoides*. This illness is characterized by tracheobronchitis that lasts about a week, with rapidly changing pulmonary shadows on radiography and a marked eosinophilia in the blood.

Heavy intestinal infections may cause abdominal discomfort and diarrhoea, but this is uncommon. The more usual feature is an iron-deficiency anaemia.

Laboratory diagnosis involves finding hookworm eggs in the stools. Chemotherapy with mebendazole is usually effective.

Preventive measures are adequate sanitation and wearing shoes.

Anthrax

Anthrax, a zoonosis, has the distinction of being the first microbial disease to be prescribed (Category B1). It must also be notified. It is now rare in the UK and Western Europe but common in Africa, India and the East where it is responsible for fatal septicaemia in cattle, sheep, dogs, camels, buffaloes and various wild animals. The causative organism is *Bacillus anthracis*, a Gram-positive sporebearer.

When wild animals die of anthrax their remains, containing spores of the bacillus, contaminate soil and vegetation. Living animals become infected by eating the vegetation; the organism enters their blood stream through lesions in the mouth.

Anthrax may be acquired through occupational or non-occupational activities. Occupational anthrax occurs mostly among people who handle wool. It may manifest with pulmonary symptoms ('wool-sorter's disease'), or cutaneous lesions ('malignant pustule'). The risk of infection is greatest from degreased wool and many infections have been acquired in carding departments where the wool is degreased and fluffed up. Other workers at risk include those who handle animal hairs, bristles and hides and bonemeal, all of which, especially if imported, may contain *B. anthracis* spores (but see below).

Pulmonary disease is caused by the inhalation of spores. These penetrate to the lower trachea, main bronchi or bronchioles resulting in an inflammatory lesion, involvement of the lungs, effusion into the pleural and pericardial cavities, possibly septicaemia and meningitis. Mortality was high but has been substantially reduced by early chemotherapy, usually with penicillin.

'Malignant pustules' result from spores that enter the body through (often inapparent) skin lesions. A small papule forms, developing into a blister in 18–48 hours and later into a large pustule with central necrosis. This may be surrounded by vesicles containing sero-sanguinous fluid. Some particularly toxic strains of *B. anthracis* may cause massive oedema (malignant oedema), extending far beyond the pustule.

Occupational anthrax occurring in non-industrial settings usually takes the form of malignant pustule in shepherds, farmers, knackermen, veterinary surgeons and butchers.

Splenic involvement, sometimes called spleen disease or Milzbrand, is an uncommon complication of anthrax.

Until recently the most common source of infection in the UK was imported bonemeal, often prepared from the bones of animals that had died of anthrax. Disinfection of bonemeal and decontamination of horns, hair and hides before they are sold and processed, and the proper use of protective clothing reduced the likelihood of infection of workers.

In the UK disease in animals and humans is controlled by the provisions of the *Anthrax Prevention Order, 1971* and subsequent amendments [*Anthrax Prevention Act 1919 (Repeals and Modifications) Regulations 1974*]. All infected animals are buried at least 6 feet deep to avoid earthworm activity which might bring spores to the surface. Human infection is prevented under the regulations which require that all imported wool, hairs, hides, etc. must pass through factories approved by the HSE where they are disinfected.

There is a vaccine for protecting sheep, cattle, horses and other domesticated animals. A different vaccine is available for people at high risk (see Chapter 7).

Laboratory diagnosis in humans is by culture of sputum from cases of pulmonary disease and pustular matter from cutaneous infections. The usual chemotherapeutic agent is penicillin. Tetracyclines and erythromycin are also effective.

Aspergillosis

The inhalation of aspergilli may result in allergic manifestations (asthma and allergic bronchial aspergillosis), aspergilloma or disseminated aspergillosis. Aspergilli may infect the outer and middle ear, paranasal sinuses and the lung. There are different presentations of disease due to aspergilli.

Aspergilloma may follow the inhalation of spores of *Aspergillus fumigatus* and *A. clavatus* (see also Microbial allergies, Chapter 6). Those at risk are farmers and people who handle mouldy hay and composts. The main feature is a ball of fungal mycelium within a cyst, arising from previously damaged lung tissue. The radiological picture characteristically shows a rounded opacity with a halo effect. Antifungal therapy is of limited value and lesions may require surgical resection.

Cases of allergic bronchial aspergillosis present with eosinophilia and increased IgE antibodies in those with pre-existing asthma. The fungus is found in mucous plugs in dilated bronchi but does not invade the tissue. The bronchial wall and the alveoli contain many eosinophils. The symptoms are those of obstructive airway disease—wheeze and cough, and often with fever and malaise. Cough results in the production of mucous plugs containing fungal mycelia. Eventually, bronchiectasis with the production of copious, purulent sputum develops. Corticosteroids have been used to clear the pulmonary infiltrates and to alleviate asthmatic symptoms.

Invasive aspergillosis occurs in immunocompromised patients. The fungus spreads through the lungs and to other organs. Pulmonary effects include haemoptysis and acute pneumonia. Nosocomial infections and 'pseudofungaemia' are often related to building and renovation activities in and around hospitals (Dewhurst *et al.*, 1990; Hruskewycz *et al.*, 1992; Goodley *et al.*, 1993). Laboratory diagnosis involves microscopy and culture of sputum and serology (precipitin) tests with patients' serum and known antigens.

Bacillary dysentery (shigellosis)

The various forms of bacillary dysentery must be notified. Two are of occupational interest. Sonne dysentery, caused by *Shigella sonnei*, is mainly a disease of young children who mix with others in day and similar nurseries. Clinically, it is mild and indistinguishable from gastroenteritis. Flexner dysentery, caused by *S. flexneri*, was once very common in institutions, especially those caring for the mentally ill. Both diseases are transmitted by the faecal-oral route, directly or by fomites. Those at risk are: (Sonne), nursery nurses and school teachers; (Flexner), mental health nurses.

The incubation period is 2–4 days, leading to illness lasting a few days and characterized by diarrhoea (bloody in about a third of cases) and abdominal tenderness. Dehydration and shock may occur in infants and the elderly. The disease may occasionally become chronic, resembling ulcerative colitis. Excretion of the organisms may continue for a few weeks after resolution of the illness.

Laboratory diagnosis is by culture of stools. Control is by personal and institutional hygiene. Antibiotics are not normally prescribed. Anti-diarrhoeal agents may prolong the carrier state and their use should be restricted as far as possible.

Brucellosis

Brucellosis is a zoonosis and is a prescribed disease (Category B7). About 200 cases are reported annually in the UK, but most are not occupation-related. The agent is the cause of contagious abortion in cattle and undulant fever in humans. In the UK the causative organism is usually *Brucella abortus* but *B. suis*, which infects pigs, may also be responsible for disease in humans. (*Brucella melitensis*, responsible for Mediterranean fever, and associated with the consumption of raw goat milk, is not found in the UK except as an imported or laboratory-acquired infection).

Farmers, veterinary surgeons, slaughterhouse workers and meat handlers are at risk. In farmers and veterinary workers infection may result from inhalation of heavily infected aerosols from birth fluids or contact of these with abraded skin or the conjunctivae. Accidental self-inoculation with the live S19 vaccine is also a hazard (Collins, 1993). Slaughterhouse workers and other meat handlers may also become infected by contact with abraded skin. Brucellosis, usually associated with *B. abortus*, is high on the list of laboratory-acquired infections, including brucella conjunctivitis.

Acute brucellosis has an incubation period of 2–7 weeks, but may be delayed. The symptoms include prostration, fluctuating fever, sweating, headaches, insomnia and backache. There may be lymphadenopathy and enlargement of the spleen. Recovery takes 2–4 weeks. In chronic brucellosis these symptoms may be complicated by endocarditis and spondylitis, the latter often causing severe sciatica and suppurative arthritis of the large joints. The condition may persist for months, with relapses. Recovery leads to immunity, although reinfection may cause a mild febrile disease.

Brucella allergy also occurs. Soon after contact with infected material a rash may develop, accompanied by transient fever and arthralgia.

Laboratory diagnosis is by blood culture and serological tests. Tetracyclines and cotrimoxazole are the usual chemotherapeutic agents.

In the UK brucellosis in cattle is controlled by an efficient vaccination and eradication scheme.

Cat scratch fever

This is also known as benign lymphoreticulosis. Local lesions develop after a history of cat scratches and may be followed by granulomatous enlargement of the regional lymph nodes which may undergo necrosis. The skin lesion develops 1–2 weeks after the scratch and lasts 1–4 weeks. Lymph node enlargement is evident 2–3 weeks after the scratch and persists for 2 weeks to 2 years. There may be mild constitutional symptoms. The aetiological agent is not known, but *Rochalimaea* spp. are suspected (Tompkins and Steigbigel, 1993).

Tetracycline is effective in some cases.

Chlamydiosis

See Ornithosis (avian chlamydiosis) and ovine chlamydiosis.

Creutzfeldt–Jakob disease (CJD)

See Transmissible spongiform encephalopathies.

Contagious pustular dermatitis

See Orf.

Cryptosporidiosis

Infected calves (i.e. with 'scours') shed large numbers of oocysts in their faeces. Lambs and dogs may also be infected. Human infection may follow as a result of contact with these animals. Sewage and then drinking water may become contaminated (Departments of Environment and Health, 1990). Transmission is by the faecal-oral route. The incubation period is 1–10 days. In humans there is a mild to profuse watery or mucoid diarrhoea and abdominal cramps, lasting 1–2 weeks.

Angus (1983) has reviewed cryptosporidiosis in humans, animal and birds. There have been major waterborne outbreaks of the disease in the United States and also incidents in the UK (Casemore, 1990). Cryptosporidiosis is an important complication of immunosuppression, as in HIV infection. Laboratory diagnosis is by microscopical examination of faeces.

Cutting oils

See Metal-working fluids.

Cysticercosis

See Tapeworms.

Cytomegalovirus infection

The cytomegalovirus is a member of the herpes group of viruses. *In utero* infections may occur, resulting in a destructive encephalopathy.

About 20% of babies acquire this agent during their first year and up to 50% of adults may be symptomless carriers of the virus which is present in the saliva and excreted in urine and other body fluids (Tookey and Logan, 1994). Infections acquired after birth are not usually symptomatic although an illness resembling influenza or infectious mononucleosis (glandular fever) may occur, particularly in immunosuppressed patients.

Pregnant women should not be exposed to large amounts of this virus, e.g. in laboratory work, as there is a risk of congenital defects in the child. Brady (1986) discussed the occupational risks for healthcare workers and concluded that although risks of exposure are unavoidable, they are not great. Tookey and Logan (1994), however, concluded that day-care staff looking after young children are at risk.

Laboratory diagnosis involves tissue culture of saliva (throat washings), urine and stools.

Dermatomycoses

See Ringworms.

Erysipeloid (the 'Rouget' of Rosenbach)

Erysipeloid is the name given to human infection by the organism *Erysipelothrix rhusiopathiae* which causes swine erysipelas (not to be confused with erysipelas in humans, which is caused by streptococci). There is pig-to-pig transmission, but direct transmission from pigs to humans is rare. Other animals are also subject to infection. In humans it is usually acquired by direct contact with animals (including bites), their hides and pelts and also with fish and shellfish. The organisms enter the human body through skin abrasions and lesions.

The incubation period is 2–7 days and the lesion that develops at the site of infection (usually the hand or forearm) is a sharply defined, elevated, purplish red zone that extends peripherally, with central resolution. There is usually burning pain and itching. Lymphangitis and lymphadenitis may ensue, and also arthritis of finger joints. Recovery usually occurs within 2–3 weeks but, rarely, disseminated skin lesions, septicaemia and endocarditis may develop (Gorby and Peacock, 1988). Infection does not confer immunity.

Laboratory diagnosis is by culture of aspirated fluid or excised tissue. The condition may be treated with penicillin or erythromycin.

There is no known method of control other than wearing gloves (where practicable).

Escherichia coli gastroenteritis

Although many serotypes of *Escherichia coli* are commensals in the human bowel about eight serotypes (the 'enteroinvasive' strains) produce toxins similar to those of dysentery bacilli and the resulting disease resembles shigellosis. In other cases there is a severe watery diarrhoea, as in cholera, which may cause dehydration. These serotypes are responsible for gastro-enteritis, especially in children, and are also incriminated in traveller's diarrhoea.

Transmission is by the faecal-oral route, either directly, by fomites or contaminated food. Those at risk are healthcare workers, especially nursery nurses, and travellers abroad. The incubation period is usually 24–48 hours.

Laboratory diagnosis is by culture of stools.

There appears to be no effective antimicrobial treatment but bismuth subsalicylate may relieve symptoms.

Eye infections

Apart from infections secondary to injuries, e.g. by opportunistic pathogens such as *Pseudomonas aeruginosa* and fungi (usually following trauma or associated with foreign bodies), at least seven infections may be acquired from the environment or animals.

Acanthamoeba keratitis (Kilvington and White, 1994) may result from exposure to the amoebae in rivers, ponds, swimming baths, hydrotherapy pools, spas and spray from water cooling towers.

Laboratory diagnosis is by co-culture with *E. coli* of corneal scrapings (swabs are unreliable). Treatment is usually with propamidine isethionate, ketaconazole and itraconazole.

Trachomatis inclusion conjunctivitis may also be acquired from swimming pools, etc. (as above), as may *Toxocara* and *Toxoplasma* infections.

Newcastle virus, present in the respiratory secretions and faeces of poultry, may be transmitted to humans and cause conjunctivitis as well as other symptoms.

'Shipyard eye', which occurs among dockers may be caused by adeno-viruses and a variety of other organisms and by exposure to organic dust (Anon., 1981). Adenoviruses, notably types 7 and 8 are known to cause acute conjunctivitis.

Improperly disinfected contact lenses are a source of eye infections (Loriot and Tourte, 1990), especially by *P. aeruginosa*.

Contact lenses should not be worn during swimming, professional or recreational participation in water sports. Micro-organisms from the water may may penetrate between the lens and the eye and initiate an infection.

Food poisoning

Food poisoning must be notified. It is included here because under certain circumstances it may be an occupational disease. There are several causative organisms, with differing symptoms and associated with different foods. They are summarized in Table 2.9 (p. 20).

Giardiasis

The protozoan responsible for this condition is *Giardia lamblia*, the cysts of which are frequently found in sewage-contaminated waters (Heap and McCullough, 1991), even occasionally in treated drinking water (West, 1991). Travellers to tropical and subtropical regions are at high risk of infection. Once acquired, infection may be spread from person to person (especially in child care) by the faecal-oral route. The main symptoms, which occur about 2 weeks after infection, are intermittent diarrhoea, anorexia, discomfort and flatulence.

Acute giardiasis usually resolves within 2–3 months but a chronic form, with intermittent symptoms, may last for years and often causes intestinal malabsorption.

Laboratory diagnosis is by microscopy of stools and treatment is usually with metronidazole.

Glanders

Glanders (also known as farcy) is a zoonosis and a prescribed disease (Category B2) although it is now very rare in humans in Europe.

A disease of equines, especially horses, it is caused by *Pseudomonas mallei* (also known as *Loefflerella mallei*). Humans acquire the disease through skin abrasions and wounds by contact with infected animals or horsehair. People at risk are equestrians, stable staff, knackers and veterinary surgeons. Laboratory staff who handle *P. mallei* are at a very high risk of infection and human-to-human transmission has been described.

Acute glanders in humans has an incubation period of 2–4 days. There is general malaise, headaches, joint pains and anorexia. Nodular abscesses form along the lymphatics and painful ulcers develop. There may be eruptions on the facial areas; erythematous patches become pustular and ulcerate. There is bone destruction and a purulent discharge from the skin or nasal lesions. The disease may pursue a chronic course, leading to lung abscesses, pleural effusion and emphysema. If it is not treated (tetracyclines, chloramphenicol) mortality may be as high as 90%.

Laboratory diagnosis (rarely attempted nowadays because of the risk of laboratory-acquired infection) is by culture of blood, sputum or pus.

Glanders is no longer a public health problem in the UK as infected animals are destroyed.

Hantavirus infections

Hantavirus infections (hantavirus pulmonary syndrome, haemorrhagic fever with renal syndrome; Korean haemorrhagic fever), is not uncommon in the Far East and has recently been reported in the USA (Bennett and Hart, 1994; Centers for Disease Control (CDC, 1993, 1994)). It has also occurred in Europe (Grist, 1988; Anon., 1990, Pether *et al.*, 1993). Various wild rodents are known to be reservoirs; the virus (a bunyavirus) is shed in the saliva, urine and faeces but there is no evidence of arthropod transmission. Human-to-human transmission is not recorded. Serious laboratory-acquired infections have been reported (Collins, 1993).

Those at risk include sportspeople, farmers, sewage workers and others engaged in outdoor activities.

Laboratory diagnosis is complex and a virologist should be consulted.

Helicobacter infections

Helicobacter pylori, a pathogen which has attracted much interest recently because of its association with gastric disorders, has been found in dental plaque; it may therefore be dispersed in aerosols created during dental treatment and inhaled by dental surgeons. Malaty *et al.* (1992) found serological evidence of helicobacter infections in dental care staff.

Laboratory diagnosis usually involves the culture of biopsy material, serology and tests for salivary antibodies, a urease test which may be done in the endoscopy room, and the ^{13}C or ^{14}C breath tests. Standard therapy includes colloidal bismuth citrate, metronidazole and either amoxycillin or clarithromycin. For an update on *H. pylori* infections see Patel *et al.* (1995).

Helminthiasis

See Ankylostomiasis, pinworm, tapeworm and *Toxocara* infections.

Hepatitis

See Viral hepatitis.

HIV infection

Apart from those engaged in prostitution, the risk of occupationally acquired infection with the human immunodeficiency virus (HIV) is low (Heptonstall *et al.*, 1993) and cases so far reported have resulted from accidental inoculation of, or exposure of mucous membrane or skin to, freshly drawn blood. In some of these cases the affected individuals have had a history of dermatitis or chapped hands. The first case of accidental HIV transmission from a patient to a nurse was reported in 1984. This followed a needlestick injury.

Healthcare workers are at obvious risk, and the occupational subgroups reported include nurses, phlebotomists and laboratory workers. Police officers may also be exposed. By September 1993, 64 documented cases of seroconversion and 118 cases of possibly acquired HIV infection among healthcare workers had been reported, mainly from developed countries (Heptonstall *et al.* 1993). Nevertheless, in view of the disastrous consequences, the possibility of occupationally acquired infections must not be overlooked. Adequate training and instruction have been advocated for healthcare workers who deal with blood, body fluids and sharps in the course of their work (BMA, 1995b). There is an extensive bibliography on this subject (e.g. WHO, 1988, 1989; UK Health Departments, 1990a).

Hydatid disease

This serious zoonosis is a prescribed disease (Category B13) but is rare in the UK. Humans are incidental intermediate hosts of the agent *Echinococcus granulosus*, the definitive host being the dog with the normal intermediate host being the sheep. The hydatid ova are passed in the faeces. If they are ingested by humans the embryo enters the portal circulation and cysts develop, principally in the liver and lungs.

Diagnosis is by X-ray, including computed tomography, to detect the cysts in the liver, lung and other organs, and laboratory complement fixation and enzyme linked immunosorbent assay (ELISA) tests. There is also a skin (Casoni) test. Treatment usually involves surgical removal of the cysts and/or administration of mebendazole.

Control is by good kennel hygiene.

Legionnaires' disease

In the UK about 200 cases of legionellosis are reported annually to the Communicable Diseases Surveillance Centre (UK Health Departments, 1988a). Although the disease mostly affects passers-by and others who work in the vicinity of the source of the organisms—*Legionella* spp, usually *L. pneumophila*—it may, under some circumstances, be claimed to be occupation or leisure related. The first documented outbreak occurred in 1976 at an American Legion convention in Philadelphia. An outbreak due to inhalation of shower mists has been reported (Anon., 1988) and one associated with aerosols from a jacuzzi (Goldberg *et al.*, 1989). Legionellas have been found in potting composts (Crawford and Grant, 1994).

In the absence of good maintenance, and if the temperature is suitable (25–42°C) the micro-organisms multiply in reservoirs of the cooling towers of air-conditioning systems, usually in the biofilms attached to surfaces. They may be associated with amoebae and blue-green algae. They are dispersed into the atmosphere in aerosols that are vented to atmosphere. These aerosols may enter premises through open windows or be captured by other air-conditioning systems. Other sources of aerosols are humidifiers, hot water systems, showers, fire sprinkler systems, ornamental fountains, spas (jacuzzis), industrial cooling waters and respiratory therapy equipment (Bartlett *et al.*, 1986). Inhalation of aerosols containing the organisms may initiate the disease. For full details see Bartlett *et al.* (1986).

The initial symptoms are an influenza-like illness, dry cough and mental confusion; later chest X-rays show consolidation. Legionnaires' disease may be serious, requiring intensive care. Treatment is with erythromycin, with the addition of rifampicin for serious cases.

Laboratory diagnosis is by culture of sputum and bronchial secretions. Serological tests may detect specific antibodies although they are less useful in the early stages of infection.

Growth and dispersal of the causative organism is prevented by good maintenance and disinfection. Plant maintenance is covered by the *Notification of Cooling Towers and Evaporative Condensers Regulations 1992* and there is an approved code of practice. See HSE (1991a, 1993d).

Leptospirosis

Leptospirosis is a zoonosis and is a prescribed disease (Category B3). It must be notified. About 100 cases are reported annually in the UK but not all are occupation or sport related.

The causative organism is *Leptospira interrogans*, of which there are 130 serotypes within 18 serogroups. The serovars *icterohaemorrhagiae, hebdomadis* and, rarely, *canicola* occur in the UK.

Rats and mice are the principal hosts of the serogroup *icterohaemorrhagiae;* hence those at risk are workers who are in contact with contaminated water: sewermen, river and canal workers, miners, those who engage in water sports and pet owners. The organisms can survive for up to 14 days in river water and may concentrate in stagnant water.

The *hebdomadis* serogroup infects cattle, field mice and voles. Farmers and, to a lesser extent, river workers are at risk.

The *canicola* serogroup infects dogs, especially puppies, pigs and rodents. Children who play with infected puppies are at risk, as are pig farmers. Infections with this serogroup are now rare in the UK as a result of canine immunization. In the USA the *pomona* serogroup appears to be responsible for infections among meat inspectors (Tobie and McCullough, 1961).

The organisms usually enter the human body by cuts and abrasions on the skin but the conjunctivae and nasopharynx are also portals. The incubation period is 7–10 days. The general symptoms of infection with the three serogroups are similar but may differ in severity. There are two overlapping phases: leptospiraemia and leptospiruria. Leptospiraemia is accompanied by malaise, severe headache, myalgia, arthralgia, sore throat, conjunctivitis and abdominal pain. The leptospires appear in the urine during the leptospiruric phase. Meningitis may develop during the leptospiruric phase.

'Weil's disease' is a label given to severe leptospirosis, characterized by jaundice, anaemia, haemorrhages, renal damage and circulatory collapse. It is usually caused by the *icterohaemorrhagiae* serogroup although other pathogenic serogroups are sometimes incriminated.

Canicola fever, associated with the *canicola* serogroup, may cause a mild meningitis.

Laboratory diagnosis is by dark-ground microscopy of blood, culture of blood and urine, and serology.

Chemotherapy is usually by penicillin, tetracyclines and/or streptomycin but this is controversial.

Control, apart from rat destruction, is assisted by wearing protective clothing, commercially laundered, rather than home washed and provision of good personal washing facilities. Workers at risk should be issued with HSE 'carry cards' which should be shown to their doctors if they report sick. These cards will alert the examining physician to the possibility of leptospirosis if the clinical features are present.

The World Health Organization (WHO, 1982b) issues guidelines for the prevention of leptospirosis. In the UK it was the subject of an 'update' by Ferguson (1991); see also Ferguson (1993) and Malone (1994) who have reviewed the zoonotic implications of nursing infected animals.

Listeriosis

Listeria monocytogenes, the causative organism of listeriosis, infects a variety of farm animals, and is present in grass silage and mouldy hay, as well as in unpasteurized milk products (especially soft cheeses).

It is responsible for an influenza-like illness in humans, with pharyngitis, diarrhoea and generalized pains. Septicaemia may lead to meningitis. The disease is often benign but there is a high mortality among neonates and the elderly. A recent report (McLaughlin and Low, 1994) indicates that cutaneous listeriosis is an occupational hazard of stock workers and veterinary surgeons who may acquire the infection, usually on the arms, from the amniotic fluids of aborted cows. Although usually mild, fever and meningitis are mentioned.

Laboratory diagnosis is by blood culture. Therapy is based on penicillin, ampicillin and related antibiotics. Sulphonamides, tetracyclines and chloramphenicol may be effective.

Louping ill

Louping ill is a zoonosis caused by a flavivirus. It is a disease of sheep, possibly tickborne, but is transmissible to humans by contact, e.g in sheep dipping, in abattoirs, or, in the case of laboratory workers, by the airborne route. Human infections are termed ovine encephalitis.

In humans it manifests as an influenza-like illness, with malaise and headache, possibly meningism, ataxia, nystagmus and strabismus. It is self-limiting, with recovery in 3–4 weeks, but more serious symptoms, including encephalitis and meningitis, may develop.

Laboratory diagnosis involves examination of the cerebrospinal fluid and serological tests with paired sera.

Lyme disease

Lyme disease, named after the area in the USA where a cluster of cases was reported, is caused by *Borrelia burgdorferi*. This spirochaete infects wild and farmed deer and wild rodents. It is transmitted from deer to deer and deer to humans by ticks (*Ixodes* species). The ticks also live freely in vegetation, hence foresters, farmers, land workers and ramblers are at risk.

There have been some 500 cases of Lyme disease in the UK since 1985. It is a non-specific illness, followed by skin lesions (erythema migrans), with neurological and/or cardiac complications.

Laboratory diagnosis is by serological examination of paired sera for antibodies (Cutler and Wright, 1994), and culture of blood, cerebrospinal fluid and synovial fluid.

Lymphocytic choriomeningitis

This is a zoonotic disease of mice, caused by an arenavirus. It is responsible for aseptic meningitis in humans. The likely mode of infection is the inhalation of dust containing mouse faeces.

Laboratory diagnosis is by tissue culture of cerebrospinal fluid, throat washings and urine.

Metal-working fluid (cutting oil) infections

Cutting oils, oil and water emulsions, are used in metal-working industries for lubricating and cooling machine tools. The oils are often recirculated and rapidly become contaminated with organisms such as *Pseudomonas, Proteus, Staphylococcus* species and coliforms. These organisms may enter the human body through cuts and abrasions, e.g. on the hands, and initiate suppurative lesions.

Inhalation of aerosols—'oil mists'—may result in allergic reactions and respiratory distress (Robertson *et al.*, 1988; Glass, 1989: Travers Glass *et al.*, 1989; Crook, 1992). Metal workers, particularly lathe operators, are at risk. Laboratory diagnosis involves culture of material from lesions.

Milker's nodule

This is a zoonosis. Infection by the paravaccinia virus (which is related to the orf virus) causes vesicles on the teats and udders of cows. Human infection arises by contact with these lesions. It presents as an isolated maculopapular lesion or pustular nodule which is mild and self-limiting.

Laboratory diagnosis is by tissue culture of material from the lesions.

Mycobacteriosis

Mycobacterioses are diseases caused by mycobacteria other than tubercle bacilli.

Swimming pool granuloma, fish fancier's finger, or fish-tank granuloma, occurs among aquarists and swimming pool granuloma among water sports enthusiasts (Collins *et al.*, 1984). Both are caused by *Mycobacterium marinum*. The organisms multiply in the water, sometimes on surfaces that are not easily cleaned, enter the human body through minor cuts or abrasions on the fingers of fish fanciers and the knees and elbows of swimmers as they climb out of the water. A solitary, raised, warty lesion develops. Secondary lesions along the superficial lymphatics may occur. This is termed 'sporotrichoid spread' as a similar phenomenon occurs in sporotrichosis.

More penetrating injuries may result in tenosynovitis. Treatment may be surgical excision or chemotherapy (minocycline, rifampicin with ethambutol).

Pulmonary disease, associated with *M. avium-intracellulare* or *M. kansasii* and occasionally other species of mycobacteria, may be acquired by the inhalation of aerosols containing the organisms, as in showers. Miners with pneumoconiosis are particularly at risk if exposed to these mycobacteria in pithead shower houses (Kaustova *et al.*, 1981). *Mycobacterium avium-intracellulare* has also been found in the dust from sawdust used for animal bedding.

Two other species, *M. fortuitum* and *M. chelonae*, both found in soil, may cause skin and other superficial lesions of humans and also of cattle, when they may be transmitted to abattoir workers (Georghiou, 1980). *Myco-bacterium terrae* has caused a few infections following injuries contaminated with soil.

Laboratory diagnosis is by culture.

Mycoplasmosis

Occupational, etc. infections with *Mycoplasma* species and associated organisms are unusual, but should not be overlooked if the patient works with cell and tissue cultures, which may be infected from the animal sources of their culture media.

Symptoms include atypical pneumonia which usually responds to cotrimoxazole and erythromycin.

Laboratory diagnosis is by culture of sputum, etc.

Naegleria meningitis

Naegleria fowleri is an amoeba that lives in warm natural waters and is therefore uncommon in the UK except in very hot weather, although it may be present in warm industrial effluents. If inhaled or taken into the mouth during swimming the amoebae may reach the meninges via the olfactory nerves. They cause primary amoebic meningoencephalitis (PAME), and acute purulent meningitis with an incubation period of 2–9 days.

Laboratory diagnosis is by microscopy and culture of the cerebrospinal fluid. Amphotericin may be useful.

Newcastle disease

This is a zoonosis, also known as pseudo fowlpest, and is acquired from poultry and other domesticated and wild birds. The causative agent is a virus belonging to the paramyxovirus group (which includes the parainfluenza and mumps viruses). It manifests as a mild upper respiratory infection, often with painful conjunctivitis. Infection results from the inhalation of dust and aerosols from diseased birds and their bedding. There are about 500 cases annually in the UK.

Poultry breeders and packers, pet shop and zoo keepers, bird fanciers and laboratory animal house staff are at risk.

Laboratory diagnosis is by isolation of the virus from eye washings and blood and by serology. Treatment is symptomatic.

See also Eye infections.

Nocardiosis

Nocardia asteroides is an uncommon opportunist pathogen of cattle which may be transmitted to humans and cause a chest infection which resembles tuberculosis. Secondary brain abscesses occur.

Laboratory diagnosis is by culture of sputum.

Orf

Orf is a zoonosis, caused by a parapox virus. It is a prescribed disease (Category B12). It affects sheep, especially lambs under one year old, and goats. When it affects humans it is called contagious pustular dermatitis. There are about 50 cases annually in the UK. Workers at risk are farmers, shepherds and goat keepers.

The agent is transmitted to humans from wool, sheep carcases and from infected plants and fences. It probably enters through cuts and abrasions in the human skin, when a mild exanthematous lesion, 1–4 cm in diameter, develops. This contains fluid and pus. There is tenderness, pain, itching and perhaps lymphadenitis.

The disease is rare now that there is an efficient vaccine for the animals.

Laboratory diagnosis in humans is by the examination of paired sera.

Ornithosis/psittacosis

This zoonosis, a prescribed disease (Category B12 (a)), officially known as avian chlamydiosis, was originally termed psittacosis or parrot disease because of its early association with psittacine birds, but as other birds (over 100 species, including domestic poultry), are now known to suffer from the disease the name ornithosis is more appropriate. There are about 500 cases annually in the UK, but not all are of occupational origin.

The causative organism is *Chlamydia psittaci* which is present in dusts from feathers and dried bird faeces. It enters the human body when these dusts are inhaled. People at risk are bird fanciers, pet-shop keepers, zoo keepers, poultry workers and taxidermists.

The incubation period is 4–15 days when an influenza-like illness develops, with a patchy inflammation of the lung with a predominantly mononuclear exudate. There is fever, headache, nausea, vomiting and pneumonitis. Diagnosis is not easy, but is suggested by an exposure to birds.

Laboratory diagnosis is by examination of paired sera.

Chemotherapy with tetracyclines is usually effective and humans may recover fully or remain carriers of the chlamydia.

Ovine chlamydiosis

This is a prescribed disease (Category B10 (b)) and is also known as enzootic abortion of ewes. It is caused by *Chlamydia psittaci* and is of importance to humans in that infection during pregnancy may result in abortion (Buxton, 1986; HSE, 1993c). Pregnant women should therefore avoid assisting at lambing (Roberts *et al.*, 1967). This may be a problem in some areas, e.g. in hill farming, where the farmers' wives normally assist because alternative help is not available.

Ovine encephalitis

See Louping ill.

Pasteurellosis

Pasteurella multocida is a commensal in the respiratory tract of many wild and domestic animal species. Infected animals may transmit the organisms by bites (Francis *et al.*, 1975). Three days after a bite a local and tender swelling (pasteurella cellulitis) may develop. This may be followed by regional lymphadenopathy and fever. Arthritis may be aggravated in patients with rheumatoid arthritis. The organisms may also be present in the upper respiratory tract of some animals, and be transmitted to humans by the airborne route (Hubbert and Rosen, 1970). This can result in pulmonary infection, manifesting as pneumonia or pleurisy, particularly in people with chronic lung disease such as bronchiectasis. The liver and meninges may also be involved.

Laboratory diagnosis is by culture of material from lesions. Broad spectrum antibiotics are usually given.

Pinworm (threadworm) infection

The pinworm or threadworm, *Enterobius vermicularis*, completes its life cycle in humans. Transmission is by the faecal-oral route or by fomites, e.g. bed linen.

Young children are often infected and spread the parasites from one to another. Adults acquire the infection during child care. People at risk are therefore nursery nurses and school teachers. Pinworms do not invade tissues and symptoms are uncommon, but they may cause pruritus ani.

Laboratory diagnosis is by microscopical examination of stools, or, better, by placing a strip of cellophane tape on the perianal skin when the patient wakes up in the morning and then examining it microscopically for ova. The condition is usually treated with mebendazole and prevented by good hygiene.

Q fever

Q fever ('Query' or 'Queensland' fever) is a zoonosis and is a prescribed disease (Category B11). It is a disease of sheep, cattle and possibly goats and is caused by *Coxiella* (*Rickettsia*) *burnetii*. About 100 cases are reported annually in the UK. Although it is usually transmitted among animals by ticks, humans are usually infected by inhaling infected aerosols from birth fluids and dusts from straw and wool. Cases have occurred among infected animal waste handlers. Sheep farmers, shepherds, slaughterhouse workers (including knackermen), tanners, wool sorters and veterinary surgeons are at risk, as are laboratory workers who handle infected material.

The incidence varies according to farming and other activities; more cases occur at lambing and calving times.

The disease resembles influenza, with fever, shivering, sweating, backache, inflamed throat, possibly a cough and/or a rash. It is usually self-limiting but a chronic form with endocarditis may occur. The incubation period is related to the infecting dose but is usually 18–20 days.

Laboratory diagnosis is by the examination of paired sera. Treatment is usually with tetracyclines and cotrimoxazole.

Rabies

Rabies must be notified. The virus (a rhabdovirus) is transmitted to humans by the saliva (e.g. by bites) of infected dogs and cats and, in Europe, red foxes. The only cases reported in the UK since the 1930s were contracted abroad. The quarantine system keeps infected animals out of the UK but animal health inspectors, dog wardens and veterinary surgeons may be at risk.

Laboratory diagnosis is by microscopical examination of specially stained brain biopsies.

Rat-bite fever

There are two agents of this exotic zoonosis, both of which have rats, mice, other rodents, and sometimes cats and dogs as their hosts. *Spirillum minus* occurs in the Far East and *Streptobacillus moniliformis* in America. Both cause skin ulcers and abscesses, followed by lymphadenopathy and fever. The systemic illnesses are termed spirillary fever or Sodoku, and streptobacillary or Haverhill fever respectively.

The first responds to penicillin and the latter to tetracycline.

Laboratory diagnosis is by culture of material from the lesions.

Relapsing fever

Relapsing fever must be notified. It may be tickborne and therefore a zoonosis, or louseborne, when spread is from person to person. Tickborne relapsing fever, caused by *Borrelia duttoni*, infects pigs and wild rodents in Africa, Asia and Latin America, where it also infects armadillos. The bites of infected ticks result in fever, headaches and splenomegaly.

Laboratory diagnosis involves examining blood films for the spirochaete. Tetracyclines provide effective treatment.

Ringworms—tinea

These skin and hair infections are caused by fungal dermatophytes. Some are zoonotic.

Trichophyton verrucosum, which infects cattle, causes tinea barbae in humans (affecting the beard).

Microsporum canis, which infects dogs and cats, causes tinea capitis in humans (affecting the scalp).

Trichophyton mentagrophytes, which infects horses, is responsible for tinea corporis in humans (affecting the body).

Microsporum gypseum, a soil fungus, may be acquired by agricultural workers. This organism, as well as other keratinophilic fungi, has been found in sewage sludge and the bottom sediments of polluted rivers and eutrophic lakes (Ulfig and Korcz, 1983; Ulfig and Ulfig, 1990).

The fungal spores enter the human body through the skin and hair. People at risk are those who handle the animals: farmers, pet-shop keepers, veterinary surgeons, chiropodists, hairdressers and zoo keepers. Laundry workers who handle contaminated clothing are also at risk.

The symptoms of ringworm include loss of hair (in tinea capitis) irritant vesicular lesions, hyperkeratosis and scaling.

Laboratory diagnosis is by microscopy and culture of hairs or skin scrapings. Whitfield's ointment and clotrimazole are used in treatment.

Salmonellosis

Many animals (including reptiles and birds) are reservoirs of *Salmonella* species which cause gastro-enteritis. Infection may be by contact with the animals or with infected slurry and effluents from cattle units and piggeries.

Laboratory diagnosis is by culture of faeces. Antibiotics are not usually prescribed.

'Scrumpox'—herpes gladiatorum

Infections, often pyogenic (e.g. impetigo, Sharp and Adams, 1990), of the face and exposed parts of the body after abrasions during contact sports are a recreational hazard (Sharp, 1993, 1994). Herpes simplex virus is one cause (Shute *et al.*, 1979).

Shigellosis

See Bacillary dysentery.

Skin infections

Apart from those mentioned in this chapter a variety of other micro-organisms may infect the skin, especially if has been traumatized (Ancona, 1990), and this can occur in the course of occupations, or sports and recreational activities.

Streptococcus suis infection

Infection by *Streptococcus suis* is zoonotic and is a prescribed disease (Category B9).

The organism is responsible for disease of pigs, especially piglets. It is transmitted to humans by contact with pigs or pig meat. The organism enters through cuts and abrasions in the skin. It is now very rare in the UK (two or three cases annually). People at risk are pig farmers, slaughterers and butchers (especially while 'boning out' pork), and in those who prepare animal food from carcases, offal and meat from various animal sources.

The symptoms include skin lesions, meningitis, followed by deafness and vestibular disturbance, and arthritis. Laboratory diagnosis is by culture of material from the lesions.

Most, if not all, strains are susceptible to penicillin.

Tapeworms

The tapeworm of occupational significance in the UK is the beef tapeworm, *Taenia saginata* (infection with the pork tapeworm, *Taenia solium*, is very rare). Normally, humans are the definitive host, harbouring the segmented tapeworm. The ova, passed in the faeces, are ingested by the cow, develop into the cysticercus, which, when eaten in undercooked meat, grows into the segmented form. If, however, humans accidentally ingest the ova, as sometimes happens in agricultural activities, the cysticercus will develop in the tissues. Cysticercosis is a serious, but uncommon health hazard.

Human infection by the fish tapeworm, *Diphyllobothrium latum*, has occurred in fishermen and others in endemic areas who eat raw or undercooked fish.

Laboratory diagnosis involves examination of faeces for tapeworm segments, and, if possible, finding the head after treatment with vermifuges.

Tetanus

Tetanus, popularly known as lockjaw, must be notified. It is caused by the toxin of *Clostridium tetani*, an anaerobic Gram-positive bacillus, the spores of which are widely distributed in soil, especially that which has received faecal manures.

Humans become infected when the spores are inoculated into deep tissues by penetrating wounds where anaerobic conditions prevail.

Those at risk include agricultural workers, workers who use heavy machinery for digging earth, fieldsports people and military personnel (gunshot and shrapnel wounds).

The toxin affects the central nervous system, leading to severe muscular spasms. Unless cases are rapidly and adequately treated, the mortality rate is high.

Laboratory diagnosis is by culture of wound tissue and fluids.

Control is by immunization. Treatment is with specific immunoglobulin and benzylpenicillin.

Toxocariasis

Also known as visceral larval migrans, this is a zoonosis. The roundworms *Toxocara canis* and *T. cati* infect dogs and cats respectively. There is no intermediate host. The eggs are passed in the faeces. When ingested the larvae develop in the intestine, enter the blood stream and migrate to the liver, spleen, lungs, eyes and brain.

Infection in humans is by the faecal-oral route. Young children who play with infected animals are at risk. Nursery nurses and teachers, and also kennel and cattery staff, can become infected in the course of their work, as may park keepers and groundsmen in areas where dogs are exercised.

Laboratory diagnosis is by examination of the stools and by serology. The larval stage may be treated with diethylcarbamizine. Control is by deworming the animals and by the education of pet owners and the general public.

Toxoplasmosis

This is a zoonosis. The definitive host is the cat, which harbours the protozoan *Toxoplasma gondii*. There are various intermediate hosts, including humans.

Infection is by the faecal-oral route: contact with cats or with soil contaminated by their faeces (French *et al.*, 1970). The organisms invade the bloodstream and lymphatics and migrate to the lymph nodes, brain, spleen and eyes.

Cattery staff and those who keep cats as pets are at risk. As toxoplasmas also cause ovine abortion, pregnant women who assist in lambing are at risk (Thomas and Joynson, 1994); infections acquired during early pregnancy may be transmitted to the fetus.

Laboratory-acquired infections have been reported (Collins, 1993), although a recent survey concludes that this risk is minimal among workers even in *Toxoplasma* reference laboratories (Parker and Holliman, 1992).

Laboratory diagnosis is by serology or histology. Treatment is by pyrimethamine and sulphadiazine, which act synergistically, or by trimethoprim with a sulphonamide (e.g. cotrimoxazole).

Transmissible spongiform encephalopathies (TSEs)

These are rare, fatal, degenerative conditions of the central nervous system and include (in humans) Creutzfeldt–Jacob disease (CJD), Gerstmann–Straussler–Scheinken syndrome (GSS), kuru and (in animals) scrapie of sheep and goats and bovine spongiform encephalopathy (BSE) of cattle. Various wild animals also suffer from similar encephalopathies.

The causative agents are termed 'prions' or 'unconventional agents'. They do not have properties in common with viruses and are extremely resistant to normal sterilization and disinfection procedures.

Although epidemiological surveys have failed to find a link between occupations and CJD it has been reported in butchers, farmers and healthcare workers, although a significant excess in these occupational groups has not been demonstrated (Ridley and Baker, 1993; Sawcer *et al.*, 1993). According to the Advisory Committee on Dangerous Pathogens (HSE, 1994a) no confirmed cases of occupational transmission of TSEs have been recorded.

In view of public concern, occupational precautions, in farming, abattoirs and postmortem examinations of humans and animals, have been formulated (HSE, 1994a).

Tuberculosis

Tuberculosis must be notified and is also a prescribed disease (Category B5) if it results from occupational contact with a source or sources of tuberculous infection. As one of these sources may be animals the disease is also a zoonosis.

Although tuberculosis, especially that caused by *Mycobacterium tuberculosis*—

the human variety—is endemic it may also be acquired as a result of exposure during work. The bovine variety, *M. bovis*, can be transmitted to humans from infected farm animals, especially cows. Occupationally, the disease is acquired by the airborne route: inhalation of infectious particles in aerosols from the respiratory tract and urine of the cow.

Those at risk from the human tubercle bacillus include healthcare workers (Sepkowitz, 1994), especially those in contact with undiagnosed cases, e.g. in the elderly. A current problem is the increasing number of people infected with multidrug-resistant tubercle bacilli. The bovine bacillus is more likely to target dairy and beef farm staff and veterinary surgeons. Seafarers appear to be much at risk; silicosis and other 'dust diseases' predispose to tuberculosis.

Laboratory diagnosis of pulmonary tuberculosis is by microscopy and culture of sputum. There are standard antituberculosis drug regimens and the vaccine BCG (Bacille Calmette-Guérin) is generally available.

Traveller's diarrhoea

See *Escherichia coli* gastroenteritis.

Vesicular stomatitis virus infection

This rhabdoviral zoonosis may be acquired from vesicles in the mouth or on the teats of cattle, horses and pigs. Veterinary staff and farm workers are at risk. In humans the symptoms resemble those of a mild influenza but vesicles may appear on the lips or in the mouth. Most cases probably go undetected.

Viral hepatitis

This includes infectious hepatitis caused by a variety of agents, including those of hepatitis A (a picornavirus), B (an orthohepadnavirus), C (a flavivirus), D (unclassified) and E (a calicivirus); they are given the acronyms HAV, HBV, HCV, HDV (or Δ virus or delta agent) and HEV. Hepatitis B is a prescribed disease (Category B8) and must also be notified.

Hepatitis A and hepatitis E are usually foodborne and result from faecal or sewage contamination. There is some evidence that sewage workers are at risk from HAV infection (Timothy and Mepham, 1984; Shakespeare and Poole, 1993), but the risks to healthcare workers from exposure to faeces, e.g. of children, requires evaluation (Viral Hepatitis Prevention Board, 1994).

Hepatitis E has occurred in large outbreaks as a result of exposure to grossly contaminated water. It is usually an acute, self-limiting disease but may lead to a fulminant, often fatal, hepatitis in pregnant women (Skidmore, 1995).

The other hepatitis viruses are bloodborne. Hepatitis B is the most common; hepatitis C (formerly known as hepatitis non-A non-B) is less common; hepatitis D is caused by a defective virus and requires the presence of HBV to proliferate.

People at risk of acquiring these bloodborne hepatitis infections are those who handle or come into contact with infected blood and body fluids. They include healthcare workers, especially those carrying out invasive procedures and those working in dialysis units and diagnostic and clinical laboratories, ambulance crews and paramedical personnel. It has been reported that approximately 1% of health workers gave positive serological tests for hepatitis B—four times higher than a matched group of non-medical workers (Patterson *et al.*, 1985). Police officers, forensic scientists and clinical waste handlers, prison officers, and to a lesser extent, some other workers are at risk. See also Astbury and Baxter (1990).

Hepatitis B and C viruses enter the human body through cuts and abrasions in the skin and wounds by contaminated 'sharps', e.g. hypodermic needles, scalpels and suture needles. Infection may result from bites by patients who are carriers or cases of the disease. This is relevant in the case of staff of institutions for care of the mentally handicapped, and also the custodial services, where there may be a high incidence of hepatitis B carriers. Hepatitis B can be acquired from very small amounts of blood; the agent is known to be more infective than the HIV virus. Outbreaks of hepatitis B, resulting from infected healthcare workers, have involved sources that are e-antigen positive.

The incubation period for hepatitis B is 4–12 weeks and the symptoms include malaise, headache, fever and jaundice. The majority of cases recover without complications. Less than 1% succumb to fulminant hepatitis. One to 10% of infected adults become chronic carriers with a high risk of chronic liver disease, including hepatocellular carcinoma (BMA, 1995a). About 50% of those infected with hepatitis C virus, however, may become chronic carriers.

Laboratory diagnosis is by serology to detect hepatitis B and C markers.

There are effective yeast-derived vaccines for hepatitis B. This is administered intramuscularly in three doses (see Table 7.3, p. 107). Satisfactory immunization is confirmed by seroconversion, which occurs in about 90-95% of recipients. There is also a vaccine for hepatitis A which is not derived from human blood. Two doses of this confer antibody response in 99% of recipients. Blood-derived immunoglobulin may confer protection for up to three months in about 86% of recipents and is available for travellers, but there is a trend away from such products.

There is as yet no vaccine against hepatitis C.

Protective measures and procedures following exposure are well publicized (see Chapter 8), both for healthcare workers and laypeople (Royal College of Nursing, 1987; UK Health Departments, 1990a; Viral Hepatitis Prevention Board, 1993; Collins, 1994).

6 Microbial allergies and toxic effects

Occupation-related microbial allergies mostly affect the respiratory tract and result from the inhalation of spores of fungi, actinomycetes and other bacteria or their constituents or metabolites. Allergies may also be caused by non-microbial agents such as wheat weevils and avian proteins. When spores are involved the symptoms vary according to their size which determine the part of the respiratory tract on which they are deposited. Table 6.1 lists the sizes of fungal and actinomycete spores and the type of disease with which they are associated. Figure 6.1 also relates spore size to the type of allergy.

Extrinsic allergic alveolitis

This condition has received much attention in recent years (see Pickering and Newman Taylor, 1994). Also known as hypersensitivity pneumonitis, it is a prescribed disease (Category B6) and an example of Type III complex-mediated hypersensitivity reaction (Chapter 3). Acute symptoms may follow exposure to $> 10^8$ spores per mm^3 and chronic symptoms may be caused by exposure to fewer spores (Lacey, 1989a; Flannigan *et al.*, 1991).

The symptoms are similar in all of the following examples of extrinsic allergic alveolitis but vary in their severity. A few hours after exposure there is an influenza-like illness with malaise, dyspnoea, fever and joint pain. There may be a dry cough. The patient recovers in 3–4 days although repeated attacks may lead to pulmonary complications.

Farmer's lung

This is often due to the inhalation of spores of *Faenia rectivirgula* (*Micropolyspora faeniae*) and/or *Thermoactinomyces vulgaris*. These are present in large numbers in mouldy hay and may also be found in grain dusts. Sometimes the spores of other fungi may be implicated (Lacey *et al.*, 1972).

Table 6.1   *Fungi and actiomycetes and the type of disease caused by their spores*

	Rhinitis	Asthma	Alveolitis
Spores > 10 μm			
Alternaria alternata	+	+	
Puccinia graminis	+	+	
Spores 4–10 μm			
Alternaria alternata	+	+	
Aspergillus flavus*	+	+	
Cladosporium spp.	+	+	
Serpula lacrimans	+	+	
Sporobolomyces roseus	+	+	
Ustilago spp.	+	+	
Spores 2–4 μm			
Arthrinium phaeospermum	+	+	
Aspergillus clavatus	+	+	+
A. flavus*	+	+	
A. fumigatus*	+	+	+
A. niger*	+	+	+
A. terreus	+	+	
Rhizomucor pusillus*	+	+	
Pencillium roquefortii	+	+	+
P. camembertii	+	+	+
P. herquei	+	+	+
P. purpurogenum	+	+	+
Sporobolomyces roseus	+	+	+
Spores < 2 μm			
Aspergillus terreus*	+	+	
Faenia rectivirgula	+	+	+
Thermoactinomyces vulgaris	+	+	+

[Some names have been changed in accordance with current nomenclature.] These species are commonly released during the harvesting of grains and are present in mouldy hay and other plant materials. Where species have been identified as causes of disease, other species in the same genus should be regarded as potential causes.

Some species produce spores of different sizes.

* These also cause infections.

Reproduced from Lacey *et al.* (1972) with permission of the author, the Society for Applied Bacteriology, and Academic Press Inc.

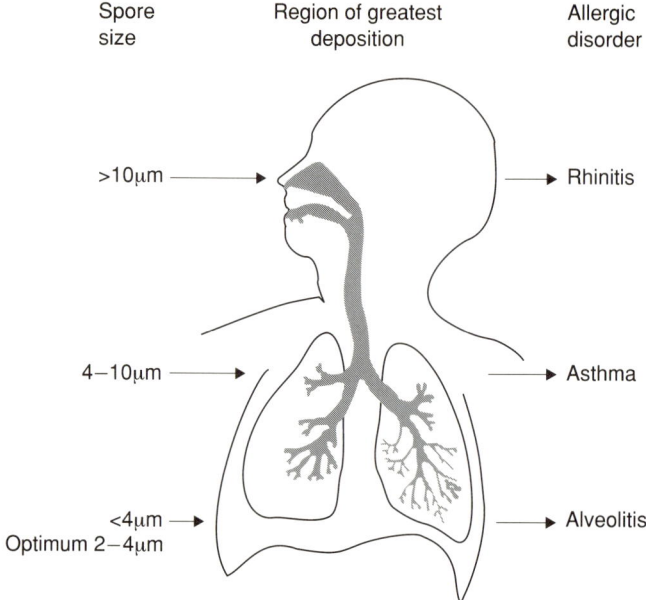

Fig. 6.1   *Spore size, region of greatest deposition and type of allergic disease. Reproduced from Lacey et al. (1974) by courtesy of Dr J. Lacey, the Society for Applied Bacteriology and Academic Press.*

Malt worker's lung

Fresh or malted barley may become contaminated with *Aspergillus clavatus* and/or *A. fumigatus* which sporulate. The spores are released into the air of the malting house when the malt is turned. If this is done by hand the malt worker may inhale large numbers of the spores (see Shi and Lei, 1986). See also grain dusts (Chapter 2), and allergies to aspergillus and 'organic dust toxic syndrome' later (this chapter).

Mushroom worker's lung

The straw used to make the compost on which mushrooms are grown commercially is degraded by various actinomycetes, especially *Faenia rectivirgula* and *Thermoactinomyces vulgaris* and mould fungi, including *Trichoderma* and *Plicaria* species. When the casing layer is disturbed, e.g. when the mushrooms are harvested, large numbers of spores are released and may be inhaled (Lacey and Crook, 1988).

In some countries the mushroom spores may be responsible for pulmonary effects. Mushroom growers who prefer growing *Pleurotus florida*, which is allowed to sporulate before picking, can be exposed to these spores. In the

UK *Agaricus bisporus* is used and is usually harvested well before sporulation (at the button stage), hence there is little or no exposure to mushroom spores (Pickering and Newman Taylor, 1994).

Cheese washer's lung

Some cheeses are inoculated before 'ripening' with a *Penicillium* species, usually *P. casei*, which is essential for the development of flavour. The moulds proliferate in the cheese and sporulate on the outer surfaces. This outer mould layer is washed before the cheeses are marketed. Inhalation of the spores during the washing process may be responsible for the allergic effects (de Week *et al.*, 1969).

Bagassosis

Bagasse consists of sugar-cane stems and foliage after expression of the syrup. It is baled and used in the manufacture of hardboards and wallboards and in soil conditioning. The actinomycete *Thermoactinomyces sacchari* (Lacey, 1989b) grows and sporulates in the bales. The spores are released into the air during milling and processing, when they may be inhaled by workers. Various fungi may also be involved. See Fink (1986).

Sewage sludge disease

This may be due to the inhalation of dust of dried or heat-treated sewage sludge, either during and after processing, or when the dried sludge is spread on land. The sludge usually contains large numbers of Gram-negative bacteria and/or endotoxins released when they disintegrate (see Endotoxicosis, later this chapter).

Potato riddler's lung

This may result from the inhalation of spores and dust (perhaps containing endotoxins) during the mechanical harvesting and sorting of potatoes (Greene and Bannan, 1985).

Dry rot lung

The spores of the dry rot fungus, *Serpula lacrimans*, are released when materials on which the fungus is growing are disturbed. Inhalation may initiate alveolitis. Dry rot lung is a potential occupational disease, although it has been described so far only in the household (O'Brien *et al.*, 1978).

Bacillus subtilis alveolitis

Like dry rot lung, this is a potential occupational allergy but, again, only household cases have been reported, as a result of exposure to wood dust containing the organisms (Johnson *et al.*, 1980). Proteases (alcalase) produced industrially from *B. subtilis* are a cause of occupational asthma.

Baker's asthma

This condition seems to be associated with the inhalation of flour which may contain spores of, e.g. *Aspergillus* and *Alternaria* spp. (Crook *et al.*, 1988). Asthma resulting from the handling, milling, transport or storage of flour is a prescribed disease (Category B7).

Humidifier fever

Humidifier fever has features similar to those of acute extrinsic allergic alveolitis. It is related to humidification systems in offices and other buildings, and the aetiological agents appear to be micro-organisms which can be grown from the water in the system, or endotoxins produced by them. A variety of micro-organisms, including bacteria, actinomycetes, fungi and protozoa, grow in the water reservoirs and recirculators of these systems. In some humidifiers aerosols are generated by spraying water on to baffles. If these humidifiers are improperly maintained, thick layers of organic growth ('baffle jelly') build up and are the source of micro-organisms distributed into the atmosphere. The organisms and their metabolites, e.g. endotoxins of enterobacteria (Rylander *et al.*, 1978; Rylander, 1981, 1986; Rylander and Haglind, 1984) are dispersed into the working areas and are inhaled by the workers.

The symptoms include malaise, fever, cough, chest tightness and myalgia. Antibodies to amoebae and other organisms have been detected, although their presence does not correlate directly with the symptoms. The onset is usually a few hours after starting work, and symptoms may abate after about 24 hours. Tolerance develops with continuing exposure, but after a few days away from the workplace, such as over the weekend or after a holiday, the symptoms may reappear following re-exposure on commencing work. Hence, symptoms often appear on Monday mornings when the air-conditioning and humidification systems are reactivated after being shut down for the weekend. Replacing spray humidifiers with steam humidifiers has solved the problem in some workplaces such as the printing industries (HSE, 1989).

Other occupation-related forms of extrinsic allergic alveolitis

These include (aetiological agents in parentheses): maple bark stripper's lung (*Cryptostroma corticale*), sequoiosis (mouldy redwood dust: *Aureobasidium pullulans*), paprika splitter's lung (*Mucor stolonifera*) and suberosis (mouldy cork: *Penicillium* spp.) (see Pickering and Newman Taylor, 1994).

'Sick building syndrome'

This syndrome consists of a wide variety of non-specific symptoms ranging from malaise, headache and fatigue to irritation of the nose, eyes, throat, skin and mucous membranes. It seems to occur in new or renovated buildings which are air-conditioned, temperature controlled, and have no openable windows. The term 'sick building syndrome' is a misnomer as it is the occupants of the building who are unwell, not the building itself. A number of people may be affected at the same time.

Although this syndrome has been associated with the use of urea-formaldehyde insulation from which formaldehyde may be slowly released, allergenic micro-organisms and/or endotoxins, the cause is still uncertain and is likely to be multifactorial in origin (Finnigan *et al.*, 1984; Gittins, 1989).

Occupational asthma

This is a prescribed disease (Category D7). Asthma has been defined by Pickering and Newman Taylor (1994) as 'Narrowing of the airways that is reversible over short periods of time, either spontaneously or as a result of treatment'. Occupational asthma occurs when the cause of the reversible airways obstruction is identified as one or more factors encountered in the workplace.

Some of the agents responsible for occupational asthma are chemical in origin. The sources of microbial allergens or the activities involved are shown in Table 6.2.

Causative organisms are mostly fungi and actinomycetes and as yet the only other micro-organism implicated is *Bacillus subtilis*, which is used in the manufacture of the proteases that are used in some detergents. The asthma is related to inhalation of the proteolytic enzymes produced by the bacillus, not the organism itself.

Not all occupational asthmas are caused by micro-organisms or their products. Other organic materials, such as resins used in soldering, sawdust from certain trees, notably the western red cedar (*Thuja plicata*), and scampi

Table 6.2   *Sources of fungi associated with occupational asthma*

Source of allergen	Fungi implicated
Cereals and grains	*Puccinia, Ustilago, Verticillium, Paecilonyces* spp.
Rotting wood	*Serpula lacrimans*
Cheese making	*Penicillium cambertii*
Food protein manufacture	*Candida* spp.
Enzyme manufacture	*Aspergillus flavus, A. awamori*
Chiropody	*Trichophytum rubrum*

protein (released when the protein in 'blown' from the shells) are also recognized causes of occupational asthma.

Allergies to aspergillus

Asthma

Eosinophils are present in the sputum. There is a Type I hypersensitivity response to aspergilli.

Allergic bronchopulmonary aspergillosis

Spores reaching the lower respiratory tract can cause an allergic alveolitis involving a Type I or Type III hypersensitivity response. This has been described in malt workers. Asthma may also be present, and chronic cough and sputum, low grade fever and eosinophilia are the main clinical features. The bronchi may be obstructed by mucous plugs containing the aspergilli. See also *Aspergillus* infections.

Allergenic and toxigenic organisms in houses

Damp conditions, rotting wallpaper and plaster, and rotting wood encourage the growth of bacteria, actinomycetes and mould fungi. The spores, endotoxins and mycotoxins of these not only affect those who live or work in the premises, but also, as a result of major disturbance, builders and demolition workers (Flannigan *et al.*, 1991). Some of the fungi may cause allergic dermatitis.

'Organic dust toxic syndrome'

First described by do Pico (1986), this is also known as 'pulmonary mycotoxicosis' and silo unloader's disease. The symptoms resemble those of allergic alveolitis: breathing difficulties, wheezing, coughing, headaches, muscular aches (Malmburg *et al.*, 1988).

It occurs among farm workers who inhale dust when they unload silos and workers at sewage treatment plants who inhale dried sludge (Rylander *et al.*, 1976). Both of these may contain large numbers of fungal spores and various micro-organisms and endotoxins (see Sewage sludge disease, p. 89). Toxic bacterial dusts are also associated with plants (Salkinoja-Salonen *et al.*, 1982) and grain silos (Pratt and May, 1984).

'Endotoxicosis'

Effects on the respiratory tract, varying from rhinitis to alveolitis, and sometimes accompanied by abdominal discomfort have been reported among farm workers and workers who handle municipal solid waste at transfer stations and landfill sites. There is some evidence that the inhalation of endotoxins, produced by a variety of Gram-negative bacilli, usually present in large numbers in such refuse, and disseminated during handling, may be responsible (Rylander, 1986; Crook *et al.*, 1987; Pickering and Newman Taylor, 1994).

Respiratory mycotoxicosis

Many fungi, notably *Aspergillus* species and especially *A. flavus*, but also *Penicillium*, *Stachybotrytis* and *Trichoderma*, produce toxic metabolites. These cause problems in the food industries, because of their toxic properties. Symptoms result when the food in which they grow is eaten (Moss, 1989), and also if it is aerosolized and inhaled (Lacey, 1989b; Flannigan *et al.*, 1991). Mycotoxins have been found in the air of flour mills (Flannigan, 1987) and are thought to be involved in building-related diseases (Sorenson, 1989; Lacey *et al.*, 1994).

Cyanobacterial toxins

Some species of blue-green algae—cyanobacteria or cyanophyta—form algal blooms on lakes and still waters in temperate climes. They produce a number of different toxins, including hepatotoxins and neurotoxins. Farm animals are often affected. Human recreational contact may be responsible for itchy, erythematous skin reactions, allergic rhinitis, asthma and conjunctivitis. Ingestion may result in gastro-enteritis (Hunter, 1991). Inhalation may result in pneumonia and pneumonitis.

7 Health surveillance and supervision

Occupational health staff

The groups of professional staff who are involved in occupational health surveillance and supervision include occupational physicians, occupational health nurses and industrial occupational hygienists.

Occupational physicians

Physicians who practise occupational medicine can now be trained and assessed for competence at two levels. At the specialist level the requirements for training include at least three years of general medical experience (general professional training) plus four years in an approved training post. During the latter period trainees often take part in formal training provided by academic departments of occupational health. This training may be full-time, day-release or by distance learning. After satisfactory assessment by examiners of the Faculty of Occupational Medicine of the Royal College of Physicians (London), Associateship (AFOM) followed by Membership (MFOM) is awarded.

At the non-specialist level, short training courses of 2–3 weeks' duration prepare candidates for the Faculty's Diploma in Occupational Medicine. This is intended for general practitioners, appointed doctors (appointed by the Health and Safety Executive), and other physicians who provide sessional advice or service to industry. It is also aimed at physicians who have an interest in occupational medicine but who intend remaining in their own specialties such as chest medicine, dermatology, clinical toxicology, public health or general practice.

The appropriate basic and specialist training programmes cover the Faculty's syllabus, which includes aspects of microbiology. This is often augmented by additional training if the physician's duties involve surveillance of workers who are exposed to micro-organisms or other biological agents.

Occupational health nurses

In the health service nurses form the major groups of occupational health professionals. These nurses are General Nurses (RGN), registered with the UK Central Council for Nursing. The post-registration professional qualification in occupational health nursing is the Occupational Health Nursing Diploma (OHND), which has replaced the Occupational Health Nursing Certificate (OHNC). In occupations where workers are exposed to micro-organisms it is desirable that occupational health nurses also have experience of infection control. In most hospitals there are close links between occupational health staff, control of infection staff, microbiologists and control of communicable disease consultants.

Occupational hygienists

Occupational hygienists may hold a master's degree in Occupational Hygiene (MSc Occup Hyg), a Diploma in Occupational Hygiene (DOH; Dip Occ Hyg) and possess either a Certificate of Operational Competence or a Diploma of Professional Competence of the British Examination Board of Occupational Hygiene (BEBOH), when they are, respectively, registered occupational hygienists or registered professional hygienists. If they are employed in microbiological or biotechnological industries it is desirable that they hold the BEBOH Certificate in the Microbiological Hazards of Occupations. In respect of occupational diseases, hygienists are usually concerned with the recognition, evaluation and control of occupational hazards in the working environment (see Chapter 9).

The professional bodies in occupational hygiene are the British Occupational Hygiene Society (BOHS) and the Institute of Occupational Hygiene. The Institution of Occupational Safety and Health covers primarily safety officers, but also has hygienists, occupational health nurses and physicians among its members.

HSE and the Employment Medical Advisory Service

The HSE employs both general and specialist inspectors who can offer advice and information within their respective fields. These specialists also have a major role in enforcing health and safety legislation. That relevant to microbiological hazards includes the *Control of Substances Hazardous to Health Regulations 1994* (COSHH) and its supporting code of practice and related documents, the *Reporting of Injuries, Diseases and Dangerous Occurrences Regulations 1985* (RIDDOR) and the *Health and Safety at Work Act 1974*.

The Employment Medical Advisory Service (EMAS) is an arm of the HSE and exists to give advice and information to both professional and laypeople on any matters relating to health at work. EMAS physicians may be contacted through the local offices of the HSE.

Laboratory services

Local hospitals and public health laboratories can offer valuable assistance and advice in the microbiological examination of specimens and samples and in epidemiological investigations.

Local authority health services

Liaison with the local consultant for communicable disease control and environmental health inspectors is also useful in the investigation and control of infections acquired during occupational, recreational and sports activities.

Health surveillance

The level of health surveillance depends of the outcome of risk assessment of the systems of work. If the risk of disease or injury is low then elaborate systems of surveillance are not warranted. All that may be required is adequate information, instruction, training for individual workers and encouraging them to report illnesses to their family doctors. Work involving moderate or high risk activities requires consideration of health surveillance by an occupational health nurse or physician. In the case of occupational infections, such surveillance may take the form of a periodic symptom questionnaire. This approach has been used for healthcare workers who are exposed to the risk of tuberculosis in the course of their work. Symptom review has replaced periodic chest X-rays in the surveillance of such staff.

Checking on immune status following vaccination or medical history of disease can also be part of the procedures for medical surveillance. Antibody levels may be checked before and after vaccination. In the case of hepatitis B, seroconversion is confirmed by testing for an adequate antibody response after a full course of vaccine has been administered.

At all levels the services of the occupational hygienist is desirable, and in higher risk situations he or she is an essential member of the occupational health service. At present, however, only a few occupational hygienists are employed by the UK National Health Service.

Pre-employment medical examinations

For employment in jobs where there is exposure or potential exposure to micro-organisms the complexity of pre-employment medical examinations depends on the level of risk involved. A simple health questionnaire may suffice. This can be checked by a physician or nurse who may then decide if further clarification of responses to the questions, and a medical examination, are necessary.

The questionnaire will include details of past history:

- previous employment—work actually done, rather than job description, as the latter may not give a good indication of risk;
- medical history, sick absences, known allergies or disabilities;
- previous exposure to physical (e.g. radiation), chemical and biological agents;
- immunization/vaccination record.

In some occupations (notably microbiological research) blood is collected so that serum may be stored (frozen) as a 'baseline' for serological tests if the worker later suffers an infection that could be occupation related. When this is done the occupational health staff should explain to the worker the reason for storing the sample and indicate which tests might be done and what benefits this may have for the individual and/or employer. This is in the light of concern about the testing of blood samples for HIV, drugs or alcohol without the individual's knowledge or consent, and the implications of such test results.

Periodic in-employment medical examinations

Instead of periodic medical examination for employees who are occupationally exposed to micro-organisms, employees are advised to report any illness and accidents at work to the occupational health department nurse who will inform the physician as and when necessary. This is important in the food industries, where skin, upper respiratory or bowel infections could result in contamination of the food, leading to food poisoning among consumers. There is little benefit in the regular examination of the stools of food handlers. Emphasis should be placed on hygiene measures by the staff at the workplace.

Special consideration should also be given to employees who intentionally work with pathogens, e.g. in microbiological, biomedical laboratories and in biotechnology.

Post-sickness examinations

Clinical review of an employee after periods of illness and before return to work may be important where there is a possibility that the sickness was a result of exposure to an infectious agent at the workplace.

Laboratory examinations

It may be necessary or desirable to test clinical specimens collected from workers or other people for the causative organisms of infections that they may have been acquired in the course of their occupations or other activities.

The containers and methods of collection are described below, together with outlines of the laboratory procedures. It must be emphasized that the success of any laboratory investigation depends, in the first place, on the proper collection of suitable specimens and samples and their prompt delivery to the laboratory. Microbiologists will give advice, and provide or specify suitable specimen containers. Only these containers should be used as others may yield unreliable results.

The types of clinical specimens are indicated by medical and epidemiological investigations. Examples of samples include throat and nose swabs, sputum, faeces, urine, blood, hair and skin scrapings.

Throat and nose swabs

Tongue depressors should be used when swabbing the throat. Both nostrils may also be swabbed. If these swabs cannot be delivered to the laboratory within two or three hours of collection the laboratory will supply swabs in tubes containing a 'transport medium' which will preserve the important bacterial flora and prevent overgrowth by other micro-organisms. Swabs are shown in Figure 7.1a.

In the laboratory suitable culture media are inoculated with the swabs and then incubated at 37°C until colonies of the organisms are visible. These are then identified by a variety of cultural and biochemical tests.

Urine

'Mid-stream' urine specimens are the most rewarding. After washing the urinary meatus some urine should be voided, the container (Figure 7.1b) filled, and the remainder discarded. If possible, 'dip slides' should also be used (Figure 7.1c). The paddle of these is coated with culture media. The paddle is dipped into the urine specimen, allowed to drain and then replaced in its

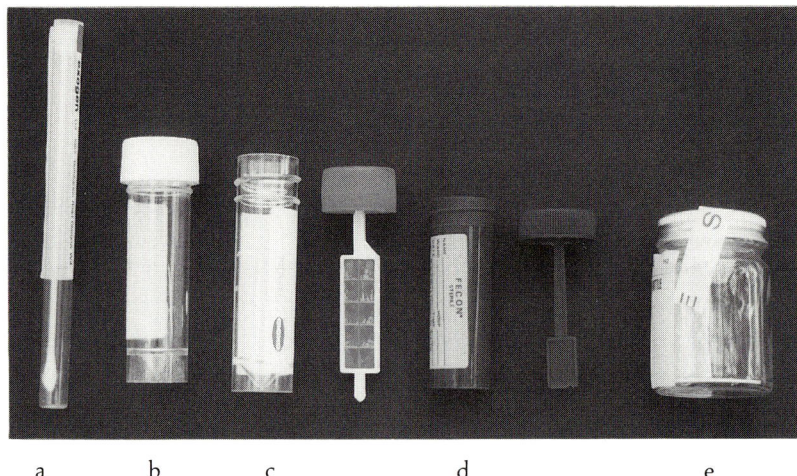

a   b   c   d   e

Fig. 7.1 *Equipment for collecting specimens: (a) nose/throat swab; (b) urine sample container; (c) dip-slide outfit for urine samples; (d) faeces container with spoon; (e) sputum container.*

container. Both the specimen and the dip slide are sent to the laboratory. The dip slide enables the microbiologist to count the number of colonies of different bacteria that develop after incubation; this helps in the assessment of their significance.

Faeces

Only a small sample is required, about the size of a pea if the stool is solid, or a small spoonful if it is fluid. A spoon is provided in or with the container (Figure 7.1d). Rectal swabs are rarely satisfactory. As faeces contain very large numbers of commensal organisms and any pathogens may be few in number special solid and liquid culture media are used to suppress the growth of 'normal' organisms and encourage that of pathogens. Colonies are identified by biochemical and serological tests.

Sputum

Sputum specimens are best collected after the patient has cleaned his or her teeth and washed his or her mouth, as the organisms of interest are those from the lung not the mouth or saliva. The material required is 'phlegm', produced by deep coughing. Containers usually have wide mouths (Figure 7.1e) to avoid soiling their outer surfaces. Laboratory examinations are similar to those from throat swabs, with, if indicated, special examination for tubercle bacilli.

Blood

Blood specimens are usually collected by physicians, nurses or phlebotomists. Proper precautions (Royal College of Nursing, 1987; UK Health Departments, 1990a) and the safe use and disposal of needles and syringes during blood collection should be stressed (BMA, 1995b) as needlestick injuries have been responsible for occupationally acquired infections.

Blood is usually taken from the antecubital vein, after applying a tourniquet to the upper arm to distend the vein and make it more prominent and easily visible. There are two standard collection techniques; syringe and needle, and vacuum tube. The skin is first swabbed with alcohol or povidone iodine.

If a syringe and needle is used the cap at the butt end of the needle container is removed and the needle placed firmly on the syringe; the needle sheath is then removed and the needle inserted into the vein. Five to 10 ml of blood are collected and the syringe emptied gently into the container without removal of the needle. Forceful squirting of the blood may result in the needle becoming detached, when blood will be distributed over the patient, operator and environment. The blood may also be haemolysed and unsuitable for some laboratory examinations. The syringe with its needle still attached is then discarded into an approved 'sharps' container (British Standards, 1990; BMA, 1995b).

In the vacuum tube method (Figure 7.2) the double-ended needle is attached to the carrier in the same way as to a syringe. The needle is then inserted into the vein and the vacuum tube pushed into the carrier so that the other end of the needle penetrates its rubber seal. The vacuum in the collection tube then ensures that the correct amount of blood flows into the tube. The tube is then removed and the remainder of the assembly discarded into a 'sharps' container.

The problem of needlestick injuries has encouraged manufacturers to develop alternatives to the standard equipment. New devices that are under test include some with retractable needles.

There are several different kinds of blood collection tubes and bottles. Some are 'plain', for the collection of blood which will clot so that the serum may be used in tests. Others contain various kinds of anticoagulants, e.g. heparin or EDTA, for use in tests on whole blood. It is important to use the correct tube or bottle.

Blood samples are subjected to a variety of chemical and serological tests to

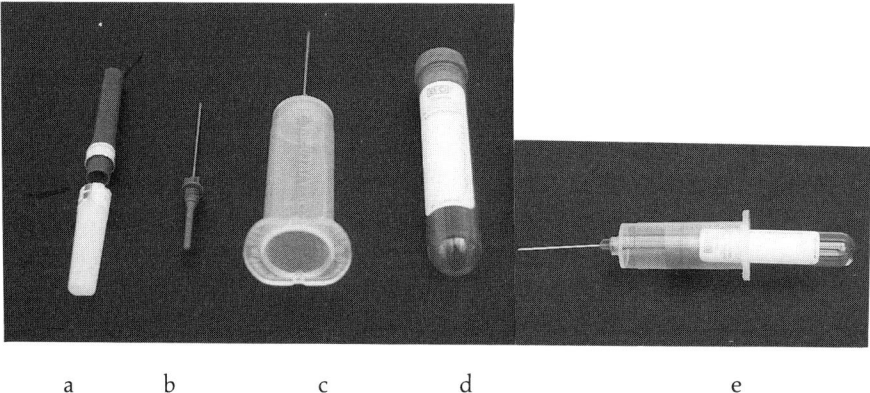

a   b   c   d   e

Figure 7.2 *The Vacutainer system for collecting blood samples: (a) double-ended needle in sheath; (b) double-ended needle exposed; (c) reusable holder, with needle attached; (d) Vacutainer tube; (e) assembly ready for use. (Becton Dickinson Vacutainer Systems, Oxford).*

detect abnormal levels of components or antibodies to micro-organisms. In microbiological tests the 'paired serum' test system is often used. The results obtained by examining 'baseline' serum (collected, e.g. at pre-employment medical examination) are compared with those from 'convalescent' serum, collected when the patient is recovering. The difference in antibody titres often indicates a specific infection.

Hairs and skin scrapings

These are necessary in the investigation of ringworm and other fungal diseases. Infected hairs are removed with forceps (and if necessary scissors) and placed in the container. Affected skin is scraped gently with a sterile scalpel, taking care not to draw blood. The scrapings may be collected on a piece of clean paper for ease of transfer to the specimen container. Gloves should be worn during the collection of such samples.

Hairs and scrapings are examined microscopically for fungi, and then cultured to confirm or identify the causative organisms.

For more detailed information about the collection and microbiological examination of human material see Shanson (1988) or Collins *et al.* (1995).

Immunization; prophylaxis

Principles of immunization

Immunization may be passive or active. In the former, antibody from an immune animal or human being is given to a person at risk of infection or disease but, as antibody has a limited life, the protection is short-lived. Passive immunization may be used prophylactically, such as for protection of travellers against hepatitis A, or therapeutically for people exposed to an infection.

Examples of the latter include the use of anti-tetanus serum for unvaccinated people suffering contaminated injuries or those occupationally exposed to rare but highly pathogenic viruses, e.g. Marburg and Ebola viruses. Serum used for passive immunization may be pooled normal serum or specifically obtained from donors whose serum is known to contain high levels of antibody to a specific pathogen. Human hyperimmune sera, when available, are preferable to those raised in animals as the latter may cause anaphylactic reactions, especially in those who have previously received serum from the same animal species.

In active immunization, the person's own immune system is activated and the protection persists for a long time. Active immunization is synonymous with vaccination, although this term originally referred to prevention of smallpox by inoculation of the cowpox virus (Latin *vacca*, a cow).

As an effective immune reaction is dependent on the clonal expansion of the antigen-specific lymphocytes, there is a delay between infection and the reaction, during which severe tissue damage leading to overt disease often occurs. This is known as the primary immune response. Fortunately, some of the expanded population of lymphocytes remain as 'memory cells' so that if the infection occurs again, the response is much more rapid—the secondary immune response. The principle of vaccination is to administer antigen which is able to induce the primary response and the generation of memory cells without causing tissue-damaging immunopathology and disease. Subsequent infection by the pathogen then generates the much more rapid and effective secondary response.

It must be stressed that no vaccine can be guaranteed to provide total protection and must never be regarded as a substitute for designated safety procedures. For detailed and comprehensive reviews of vaccines, immunization schedules, dose and routes of administration, adverse reactions, contraindications, recommendations for use and supplies of vaccines see UK Health Departments (1992) and Kassianos (1994).

Types of vaccine

The three main types of vaccine are whole killed pathogens, living attenuated pathogens and subunit vaccines. The latter include the toxoids (inactivated toxins) derived from the diphtheria and tetanus bacilli (*Corynebacterium diphtheriae* and *Clostridium tetani*) and protective antigens produced by genetic recombination, e.g. the more recent hepatitis B vaccines. The nature of the vaccines given during childhood, to travellers and to those exposed to occupational infectious hazards are listed in Table 7.1. As a general rule, a single administration of a live attenuated vaccine induces long-lasting protective immunity while several doses of the killed vaccines are required. Some live vaccines are contraindicated in immunosuppressed people including those infected with the HIV. See UK Health Departments (1992) for details.

Vaccination schedules

Immunization schedules and other prophylactic measures are designed for (a) routine use for children, (b) adults exposed to unusual or exotic infections, (c) travellers to regions where there are infectious health hazards, and (d) those exposed to infectious health hazards at work. In the UK children should be routinely vaccinated against diphtheria, tetanus, pertussis, poliomyelitis, *Haemophilus influenzae* Type B (a cause of meningitis), measles, mumps, rubella and tuberculosis. Some of these vaccines give lifelong immunity while others require booster doses later in life or before expected exposure to an agent. The schedules for adults requiring additional immunization for travel or for occupational reasons are listed in Table 7.2.

Occupational health services advise on, and often provide, vaccination. Consent for vaccination must always be obtained. Travellers may require evidence of vaccination against yellow fever (the certificate is valid from 10 days after vaccination to 10 years). Certificates for cholera vaccination are no longer officially required but countries may impose ad hoc requirements in cases of epidemics. Travellers are therefore advised to obtain certificates or they may be subjected to vaccination at border posts, with risk of infection by hepatitis B or HIV. Unlicensed vaccines for named patient use only are available against bubonic plague and tickborne encephalitis (see UK Health Departments, 1992).

An Annex to the EC Directive on the protection of workers from biological agents, etc. (European Commission, 1990) states that vaccinations should be offered where an assessment demonstrates a risk of exposure to a biological agent for which a vaccine exists. Workers should be informed of the risks of not being vaccinated.

Table 7.1   *The nature of the principal human vaccines*

Anthrax	Alum-precipitated sterile culture filtrate of *Bacillus anthracis*.
Cholera	Heat-killed *Vibrio cholerae*.
Diphtheria	Toxoid. Formalin-inactivated purified toxin of *Corynebacterium diphtheriae*. Often combined with tetanus and pertussis vaccines (DTP).
Haemophilus influenzae	Purified capsular polysaccharide conjugated to proteins, usually diphtheria and/or tetanus type B toxoids.
Hepatitis A	Formaldehyde-inactivated virus. Pooled human serum may be used for short-term protection, e.g. for travellers.
Hepatitis B	Viral surface antigen (HBsAg) prepared by genetic modification in yeasts.
Influenza	Whole virus disrupted by organic solvents or purified surface antigens. The influenza virus alters its antigenic properties regularly so vaccines must be 'tailor-made' for a particular epidemic.
Measles	Live attenuated virus. Usually combined with live attenuated mumps and rubella viruses (MMR vaccine).
Mumps	See measles.
Pertussis	Killed *Bordetella pertussis*. See Diphtheria.
Poliomyelitis	Live oral polio vaccine (OPV) containing attenuated types I, II and III viruses OR enhanced potency inactivated polio vaccine (eIPV) containing formalin-killed types I, II and III viruses (only for use in those for whom a live vaccine is contraindicated).
Rabies	Virus inactivated by beta-propriolactone.
Rubella	See measles. Single antigen vaccines are available for girls aged 10–14 years who did not receive MMR vaccine in childhood.
Tetanus	Toxoid. Formalin-inactivated purified toxin of *Clostridium tetani*. See Diphtheria.
Tuberculosis	Live attenuated *Mycobacterium bovis* (Bacille Calmette-Guérin (BCG) vaccine).
Typhoid	Heat-killed *Salmonella typhi* OR purified Vi capsular polysaccharide antigen of *Salmonella typhi* OR live attenuated *Salmonella typhi* in capsules for oral administration (Ty21a vaccine).
Yellow fever	Live attenuated virus.

Table 7.2 *Schedules for adults requiring immunization for reasons of travel or occupational risks*

Anthrax	Four doses, 0.5 ml i.m. with 3-week intervals between first three doses and 6-month interval between 3rd and 4th doses. Annual boosters.
Cholera	One dose, 0.5 ml i.m. or s.c. Boosters, 1.0 ml i.m. or s.c. or 0.2 ml i.d. every 6 months or as required for travel.
Hepatitis A	Two doses, 0.1 ml i.m. at 2–4-week intervals and a booster 6–12 months later. Pooled immunoglobulin may be given for short-term passive protection.
Hepatitis B	Three doses, 1.0 ml i.m. at 0, 1 and 6 months (or an accelerated regimen with doses at 0, 1 and 2 months, with a booster at 12 months).
Influenza	One dose, 0.5 ml i.m. or s.c.
Rabies	Three doses, 1.0 ml s.c. or i.m. or 0.1 ml i.d. at 0, 7 and 28 days. Booster every 2–3 years. Hyperimmune serum is available.
Typhoid	
Whole cell	Two doses, 0.5 ml i.m. or deep s.c. at 4–6-week interval with booster every 3 years. Second and booster doses may be given as 0.1 ml i.d.
Vi antigen	One dose, 0.1 ml i.m. or deep s.c. Booster every 3 years.
Oral Ty21a*	Three doses, one capsule on alternate days. Three-dose booster annually.
Yellow fever†	One dose, 0.5 ml s.c. Booster every 10 years

i.m. = intramuscular, s.c. = subcutaneous, i.d. = intradermal.
* Not recommended for those living in endemic areas.
† Vaccination only available at designated centres which issue certificates valid for 10 years.
Adapted from manufacturers' Data Sheets (APBI Data Sheet Compendium, 1995–96) and UK Department of Health, 1992.

Hepatitis B prophylaxis

This requires special consideration as the European Parliament has passed a special resolution (A30027/93) that employers should be obliged to offer hepatitis B vaccination to all workers who are at risk in that they come into contact with blood at least once a month. The risk assessment should be based on job function, not job title and employers should bear the cost.

Malaria prophylaxis

At present there is no vaccine against malaria, although some experimental ones are undergoing clinical trials. Chemoprophylaxis is therefore used and is recommended for travel to many tropical countries. As the type of malaria, and resistance to antimalarial agents, varies from region to region and from time to time, up-to-date medical advice on suitable regimens should be obtained.

People becoming ill after return from an endemic area should seek medical advice promptly and should give details of recent travel as a delayed diagnosis may have serious, even fatal, consequences.

International travel

Infections acquired during foreign travel may be classed as occupational or sport related if the victim is travelling on business, for sporting occasions or in the course of research or exploration. Examples of such infections are given in Table 7.3.

Occupational health physicians and medical advisers to sports and other organizations are often asked to give advice on the prevention of such infections, e.g. appropriate immunization, diet, personal precautions. Although it is already available the information needs periodical updating, otherwise advice may be contradictory (Masterton and Green, 1991), as the hazards are always changing, and 'new' diseases emerge and well-known infections occur in places where they were hitherto unknown or of little significance.

The Medical Advisory Service for Travellers Abroad ('MASTA', London

Table 7.3 *Some infections that may be acquired during foreign travel**

Cholera	Legionnaires' disease
Diphtheria	Malaria
Dysentery	Meningitis
amoebic	Paratyphoid fever
bacillary	Plague
Gastroenteritis	Treveller's diarrhoea
Giardiasis	Trypanosomiasis
Helminthiasis†	Typhoid fever
Hepatitis A, B, C	Yellow fever

* Excluding many of the rarer arthropod-borne diseases.
† Includes infections with roundworms, filarias, hookworms, schistosomes.

School of Hygiene and Tropical Medicine) and the medical departments of most airlines will provide up-to-date information and advice (on a commercial basis) about infections that are currently of concern in various parts of the world.

Valuable information for travellers, especially for those visiting tropical areas, e.g. for research and exploration, is contained in a booklet issued by the Australian National University (1990). Other useful information is given by Coralli (1985), Cossar *et al.* (1985) and the British Medical Association (BMA, 1989).

Diet

Many of the infections that affect travellers are foodborne and/or waterborne. Contamination of raw food is highly probable in some areas, as is water in rural and undeveloped areas. Table 7.4 lists foods which should be regarded as suspect and therefore avoided. Unless reliable piped or bottled water is available, all water should be boiled or otherwise disinfected. Bottled water purchased locally may be unsafe: the practice of refilling such bottles with local tap or other water and sealing them with forged labels is not unknown.

Hands should be washed thoroughly before food is handled.

Personal precautions

These depend on the geographical area visited. In areas where disease may be spread by arthropod vectors, exposed skin should be covered, especially at night, and insect repellents used. Sleeping arrangements should include mosquito netting. In damp or swampy places, where leeches may be present, legs should be covered. In bush and grassland protection against spiny or prickly foliage, which may harbour opportunist dermatophyte fungi and other micro-organisms, is also recommended. Cuts, scratches and other skin lesions

Table 7.4   *Foods best avoided during foreign travel in undeveloped areas*

Raw fish and shellfish
Raw vegetables
Salads
Fresh fruits except those with thick skin and personally peeled
Unpasteurized milk and dairy produce
Ice cream
Cold meats
Any undercooked foods

should be covered with waterproof dressings. Swimming and bathing in contaminated rivers, pools, etc. should be avoided as far as is possible.

Post-travel medical examinations

The examining physician should be alert to the possibility of a tropical disease when a traveller develops an illness after returning from Africa, India, the Far East and/or any other undeveloped area. Depending on the area visited and the presenting clinical features, microbiological examination of blood films for malarial parasites or faeces for helminths and protozoa may be indicated.

8 Minimizing exposure to pathogens

Although employers have a statutory duty (Chapter 10) to protect their employees against exposure to pathogenic micro-organisms while they are at work, employees also have a responsibility for their own health and safety. It is highly desirable that they are aware not only of any risks involved in their work but also of precautions they, as well as their employers, should take to avoid exposure. People who engage in sports and recreational activities in which there is a possibility of exposure should also be aware of the risks and precautions.

Many precautions involve personal hygiene. Information and guidance about other precautions are provided in HSE leaflets and 'carry cards' (Appendix 2) which should be issued to the staff concerned. Other publications should, where relevant, also be available to supervisors and occupational health staff.

The ubiquity of micro-organisms, even of pathogens, makes it impossible to offer comprehensive advice on the prevention of exposure. In the following sections, therefore, some appropriate precautions are outlined as recommended in the publications cited.

In addition to medical surveillance (Chapter 7), protection may be afforded by:

- personal hygiene;
- the elimination or reduction of reservoirs and sources of micro-organisms;
- prevention of dispersion and transmission;
- information and training;
- provision and wearing of protective clothing and equipment.

Personal hygiene and health care

Information about the risks of microbial diseases associated with work, sport or recreations, including the portals through which micro-organisms may enter the body, should encourage a high standard of personal cleanliness and give such basic advice as:

- wash the hands if contaminated during work;
- cover all cuts, scratches and other exposed lesions with waterproof dressings;
- seek medical advice about any illnesses that might possibly be related to work, sport or recreation.

Elimination and reduction of reservoirs and sources of micro-organisms

Globally this is an impossible task but in industry it may be achieved in several ways. Monitoring of raw materials and rejection of those that contain pathogenic organisms has become standard procedure in some organizations, notably those concerned with food manufacture. In the biotechnology industries harmless or less hazardous micro-organisms, either naturally occurring or produced by genetic modification, may be used instead of pathogens.

People who engage in outdoor sports and recreations are exposed to micro-organisms in the environment. Environmental protection regulations are contributing to the clearance and avoidance of many sources of micro-organisms, e.g. in the atmosphere, in water and in litter.

Prevention of dispersion and transmission

In industry this may be achieved by mechanically shielding workers and limiting their exposure to micro-organisms and their allergenic and toxic products. Workers may be shielded by containment of the process in closed systems and by providing exhaust ventilated enclosures (e.g. microbiological safety cabinets). The principles of containment are well documented (Frommer *et al.*, 1989, Collins and Grange, 1990; Collins, 1993).

Information and training

In industry employees should be properly informed of any health risks to which they may be exposed as a result of working with micro-organisms. This is now a legal requirement in the UK and the European Union. It follows that they should receive training in the work they will do.

The Health and Safety Commission, through its Executive and the various Health Service advisory committees, produces a number of leaflets on the hazards of various industries, including agriculture and water. These are listed in the References and in Appendix 2. Information about hazards and personal protection in sports and recreations is sketchy but several sporting organizations (Appendix 3) include warnings about infections in their general information documents (see below).

Personal protective equipment

Employers have a legal duty to provide personal protective equipment in certain industries and for certain activities; employees have a legal duty to use it.

Protective clothing

The choice of protective clothing for work with micro-organisms in industry, or where there is incidental exposure to them, must be made with regard to the places where they will be worn—indoors or outside, and of other hazards, e.g. chemical and physical, to which the worker may be exposed and which may offer a greater risk. Suitable protection for those who deliberately handle micro-organisms in laboratories, or who are exposed to them incidentally in the course of their employment, is determined by an assessment of risk. The first group may require gowns or overalls that completely cover their street clothing, including the chest area, and have tight-fitting cuffs at the wrist. These may be supplemented with plastic aprons, especially when handling blood and micro-organisms classed as 'dangerous pathogens' (HSE, 1995a).

Heavy-duty boots are necessary for outdoor work and where there is the possibility of penetrating wounds from refuse, e.g. hypodermic needles in clinical waste. Gloves vary from those with metal inserts to protect against wounds to surgeon's gloves, suitable for most laboratory work. A wide variety of protective clothing—suits, overalls, footwear and headwear is listed in manufacturers' catalogues.

Eye and face protection

Safety spectacles, goggles or visors should be selected according to the level of risk—the likelihood of splashes. The best types of safety spectacles have side-shields. Full-face visors should protect the neck as well as the face (Figure 8.1a and b).

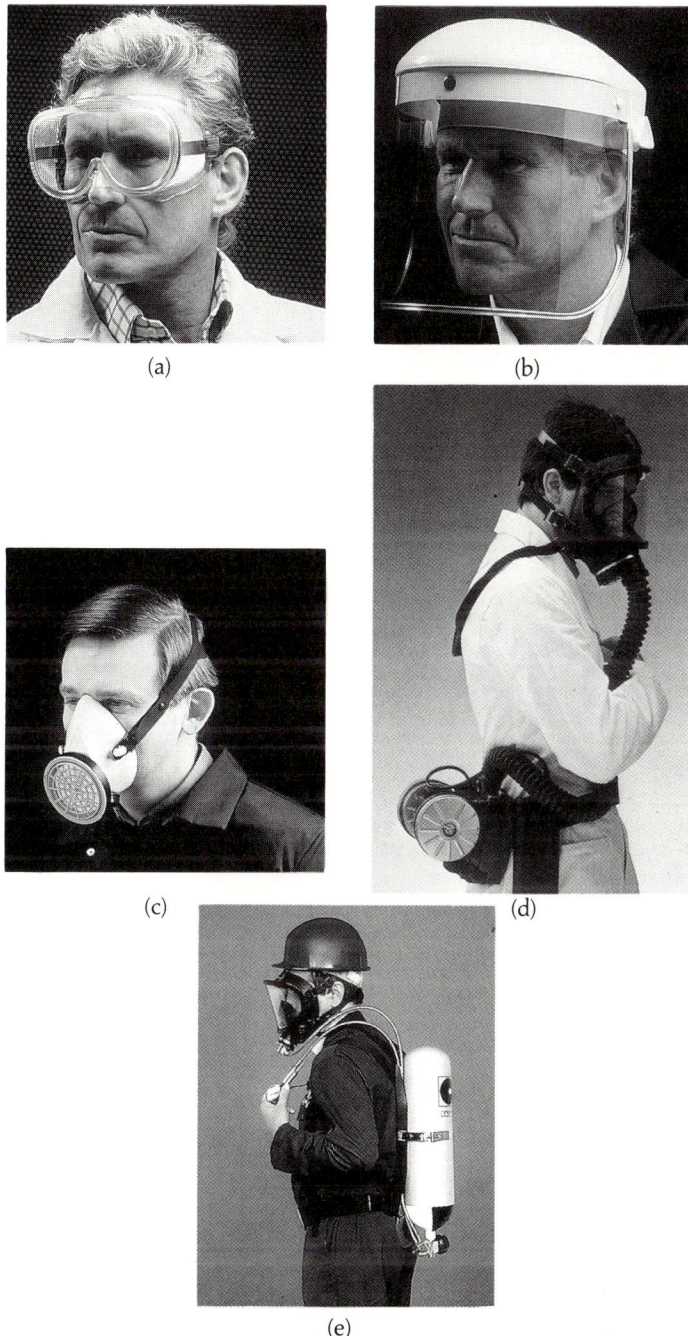

Fig. 8.1 Eye and respiratory protection. (a) safety goggles; (b) full-face visor (c) half-mask respirator; (d) powered respirator; (e) self-contained breathing apparatus. Courtesy of the Director, Institute of Occupational Health, University of Birmingham.

Respiratory protection

The risk assessment will indicate the appropriate equipment. Disposable masks, made of fibres and having soft metal parts that enable them to be moulded to the face, offer protection against the inhalation of dusts and fungal spores. Some masks fit under visors. Surgeon's masks and thin paper masks are inadequate. If better protection is necessary the half-mask respirator, fitted with a dust cartridge may suffice. The next step, suitable for protection against the inhalation of bacteria, is the full-face respirator, fitted with a high efficiency particulate air (HEPA) filter. Finally, there are powered full-face respirators, in which filtered air is ducted to the face by a battery-driven motor (Figure 8.1d and e). If full-face respirators are to be used then each must be fitted to an individual wearer and used by that person alone. The canisters for half- and full-face respirators must be the correct type—dust or HEPA. Canisters for use against chemical and vapours may not remove dust or micro-organisms (see Harrington *et al.*, 1992).

Other personal protective equipment

Some police forces provide their officers with a small kit containing (1) a pair of gloves, (2) a clinical waste bag, (3) a Layerdal personal resuscitator to place over the face of the patient during mouth-to-mouth resuscitation, and (4) an antiseptic wipe. Such a kit could be useful in other occupations.

Precautions in specific activities

Arable farming and horticulture

Work with hay, growing, harvesting and storage of grain, and crop plants (including mushrooms), and handling of malt may result in health problems that affect the eyes, nose and lungs. Some fertilizers may be infected. Workers should therefore:

- avoid creating excessive amounts of dust;
- avoid the inhalation of dusts by wearing suitable masks when indicated;
- seek medical advice about symptoms following workplace exposures, e.g. irritation of eyes, mucous membranes and any breathing difficulties.
- wear masks or other respiratory protection when spreading sewage sludge on land;
- avoid touching bone-derived and meat-derived fertilizers with the bare hands.

There are HSE leaflets on farmer's lung and grain dust (Appendix 2). See also HSE (1993a, b).

Animals and animal products

See Zoonoses.

Athletics and contact sports

Guidelines on hygiene in sports have been published by the UK Health Education Authority, the Scottish Sports Council and the Sports Council of Wales (see Appendix 3). The following precautions are suggested:

- cover all cuts and abrasions with waterproof dressings;
- avoid communal baths, use individual showers;
- do not walk barefoot on wet floors in dressing rooms and communal areas;
- avoid barefoot sporting activities;
- ensure that tetanus vaccination is up to date.

Exposure to blood

Hepatitis B and hepatitis C, possibly HIV, are the main hazards of contact with blood. Guidance for healthcare workers who are at risk from blood is given by the UK Health Departments (1990a, 1993) and the Royal College of Nursing (1987), and for other workers by Collins (1994). In summary, those who are potentially exposed should:

- treat all blood as if it is infected (it may be!);
- avoid handling any blood-stained articles with the bare hands; this includes used hypodermic needles, sanitary towels, tampons, dressings, clothing;
- cover all cuts and abrasions with waterproof dressings;
- immediately wash thoroughly with soap and water any part of the skin if it accidentally comes into contact with blood;
- immediately wash thoroughly with soap and water any prick or cut from a blood-stained article; avoid sucking the wound; seek medical attention as soon as possible;
- be immunized against hepatitis B.

Residential and day care of children and the elderly

The following precautions are recommended in residential and day-care activities and premises:

- maintain a high standard of personal hygiene;
- cover all cuts and abrasions with waterproof dressings;
- wash hands well after contact with nappies, incontinence pads, etc.,

- avoid contact with the saliva of children who may harbour cyto-megalovirus;
- inform the doctor or supervisor if pregnant or possibly pregnant;
- maintain a high standard of hygiene in the care premises; do not place too much reliance on disinfectants: cleaning with soap and water is usually, and often more, effective.

Construction work

The main hazards arise during demolition and refurbishment, and from contact with soils. Workers should:

- avoid inhaling dust during the demolition of old properties where materials may be infected with fungi and other micro-organisms;
- cover all cuts and abrasions with waterproof dressings;
- report penetrating injuries and seek medical advice;
- ensure that vaccinations, especially against tetanus, are up to date.

Cutting fluids

See Metal-working fluids.

Funerals and undertaking

Ideally, funeral directors, and morticians who engage in embalming the dead, should be notified by the medical or hospital authorities if the subject died of a notifiable infectious disease (UK Health Departments, 1988b). Cadavers received in body bags should not be embalmed unless enquiries reveal that the bags were unnecessary. When other bodies are embalmed care is needed to avoid sharps injuries, e.g. from needles and cannulas, and protective clothing should be worn for this process as well as for 'hygienic preparation' (gloves, masks, eye protection, as well as the usual gowns) to minimize contact with blood and body fluids (e.g. leaked faeces). See McDonald (1989); Nwanyanwu (1989); Healing *et al.* (1995) and Mortuary and post-mortem room staff below.

Laboratories

As indicated earlier, this subject is complex and reference should be made to specialist publications (HSE, 1991b,d, 1994b; Collins, 1993; WHO, 1993).

Legionnaires' disease

There is little that individuals can do to avoid exposure to *Legionella pneumophila* but owners and operators of air-conditioning plant have a legal duty under the *Notification of Cooling Towers and Evaporative Condenser Regulations 1992* to register their plant and are subject to inspection. They are required to conform with the Code of Practice (HSE, 1991a; see also HSE, 1993d). The requirements are too detailed to be considered here but in general they relate to proper maintenance which avoids the build-up of biofilm in which the legionellas multiply. The biofilm must be removed by adequate cleansing and growth of legionellas inhibited by treatment with an approved biocide. Treatment with biocide alone is inadequate: it may not reach the organisms in the biofilm.

Other installations, such as humidifiers, particularly those of the spray and spinning disc type, also require careful maintenance. Cold water systems in which the water is stored above 20°C and hot water systems in which it is stored below 60°C may also permit the growth of legionellas, which may then be dispersed by shower heads, etc. (Water stored at 60°C should be delivered at a lower temperature, e.g. 50°C, to avoid scalding the users.) (See Agar and Tickner, 1985; Bartlett *et al.*, 1986; Collins and Grange, 1990.)

Metal-working fluids

Health problems may result from contact of metal-working fluids with the skin and by the inhalation of mists generated during their use. There are HSE leaflets (Appendix 2). See also HSE (1992a). The following precautions are recommended:

- avoid contact with skin; apply skin conditioner after work;
- cover all cuts and abrasions with waterproof dressings;
- avoid inhaling mists;
- wear protective clothing; change it regularly; do not take dirty protective clothing home for washing;
- do not put oily rags into pockets of your own clothes;
- do not drink or smoke in the work area;
- where there is contact with these oils, have your exposed skin inspected monthly by the occupational health nurse;
- see a doctor if you have any breathing difficulties.

Mortuary and post-mortem room staff

Cadavers may be infected with a variety of micro-organisms and precautions are necessary to avoid acquiring, e.g. bloodborne diseases, skin infections, and, especially during post-mortem examinations, exposure to tubercle bacilli. Use of gloves, protective clothing, face protection and a high standard of hygiene are the most important precautions. Specialist advice is given by the UK Health Departments (1981, 1988b), Calder (1987), HSE (1991c, 1994a) and the Royal Institute of Public Health and Hygiene (1995); see also Healing *et al.* (1995).

Additional precautions are necessary during post-mortem examinations in known or suspected cases of transmissible spongiform encephalopathies (e.g. Creutzfeldt–Jacob disease). These are set out in detail by the Advisory Committee on Dangerous Pathogens (HSE, 1994a).

Offices and similar premises

Humidifier fever, sick building syndrome, etc. and legionnaires' disease may result from inhaling micro-organisms, their toxins and other organic matter (and sometimes chemical), released by improperly maintained air-conditioning systems. Prevention of such exposure is the province of employers and their engineers.

There are legal requirements for the correct maintenance of air conditioning systems. See Legionnaires' disease.

Outdoor activities

These precautions are recommended for foresters, walkers, campers, park keepers, groundsmen, hunters, etc.:

- avoid contact with animal faeces, especially those of dogs;
- wear leg protection against tick bites in wooded areas and especially where there are deer;
- guard against pricks from spiny plants;
- ensure that vaccinations, especially against tetanus, are up to date.

Refuse and waste handling

Municipal solid waste contains large numbers of micro-organisms capable of causing skin infections and endotoxins derived from Gram-negative bacilli. Building wastes may contain large numbers of spores of allergenic fungi. Clinical waste may contain bowel and lung pathogens and articles contaminated with blood, including hypodermic needles and other sharp objects. Precautions therefore include:

- cover all cuts and abrasions with waterproof dressings;
- wear heavy duty gloves and protective clothing, including boots, when removing waste:

- avoid inhalation of dusts: wear masks for dusty processes;
- wash hands if contaminated;
- do not eat, drink or smoke when disposing of domestic, industrial or clinical waste.

For further information see HSE (1993e), Collins and Kennedy (1992, 1993); London Waste Regulation Authority (1994).

Sewage and sewage sludge handling

The following precautions are recommended:

- always wear protective clothing, including gloves and boots;
- do not take protective clothing home for laundering;
- cover all cuts and abrasions with waterproof dressings;
- wash hands frequently, and especially before visiting canteens and/or eating and drinking;
- do not eat, drink or smoke while at work;
- when 'jetting' with high pressure sprays wear face visors.
- ensure vaccinations (especially tetanus, hepatitis A, poliomyelitis and typhoid fever) are up to date and seek advice about hepatitis B vaccination.

Tuberculosis

Workers who are exposed, e.g. in health care, teaching, prison custody, agriculture and care of the elderly should have BCG vaccine provided that they are tuberculin negative (Heaf or Mantoux test) and have not previously received the vaccine. Periodic chest X-rays for these workers have largely been discontinued in view of their lack of efficiency in detecting cases of tuberculosis and the undesirable exposure to X-radiation.

The British Medical Association (BMA, 1990) and the British Thoracic Society (1990) offer useful advice, as do the UK Health Departments (1990b).

Waterborne infections

The HSE issues warning cards about leptospirosis. The Amateur Rowing Association (Appendix 3) has published a Safety Code which includes advice on avoiding waterborne infections.

As leptospirosis is the most likely infection to follow exposure to polluted water precautions should be geared to minimizing such exposure. These measures will also be effective against less common waterborne infections, including those that affect the eyes:

- control the rat population where possible, e.g. by reducing available litter: 'wheelie-bins' with lids are better than open refuse containers or plastic bags;
- reduce contact with polluted water as far as possible, e.g. by wearing protective clothing; avoid immersion if possible;
- cover all cuts and abrasions with waterproof dressings;
- wash any new cuts under running water as soon as possible;
- use available washing facilities—showers, etc.
- shower or bath after contact with polluted water;
- use laundry facilities rather than wash clothing at home;
- remove contact lenses before carrying out any work where there is a possibility of contact of eyes with polluted water;
- seek medical attention if sick, especially with influenza-like symptoms that occur soon after exposure;
- ensure that vaccinations are up to date.

Zoonoses

Full protection against diseases of animals transmissible to humans is not possible except in certain kinds of laboratories.

The Health and Safety Executive issues 'Carry Cards' and leaflets for agriculture workers and about leptospirosis and BSE (see Appendix 2). There is an HSE publication that offers advice on precautions against some zoonoses (HSE, 1993c) and two that give specific advice on work with laboratory animals, especially about allergies (HSE, 1990a, 1992b).

Where possible, and certainly in the handling of sick animals, the following precautions are suggested:

- wear protective clothing;
- cover all cuts and skin abrasions with waterproof dressings;
- wash hands when contaminated;
- avoid inhaling dust from bedding, litter materials and lairages;
- avoid eye and face exposure during lambing and calving, etc.
- if in contact with farm animals read and carry HSE 'Carry Cards'.

For farm workers and others who are in contact with cows suffering from BSE the HSE leaflet suggests that they:

- wear protective clothing, gloves and eye protection;
- avoid cuts and puncture wounds;

- cover cuts and abrasions with waterproof dressings;
- wash hands after any contact;
- wash down contaminated areas with disinfectant and water;
- rinse protective clothing free of debris after use and wash with water and disinfectant.

9 Microbiological monitoring of materials and the working environment

Monitoring exposure to substances in the environment is usually the area of expertise of an occupational hygienist. Some of this work may be done with simple, direct reading instruments but detailed assessment of exposure requires laboratory analysis of environmental samples. Similarly, for micro-biological investigations involving the determination and assessment of exposure to micro-organisms some samples must be sent to a microbiological laboratory.

Scope of tests

Testing and monitoring includes:

(1) examination of raw materials or products for micro-organisms that might cause disease;
(2) monitoring the environment for such micro-organisms or for evidence of their presence.

Raw and process materials

These materials are examined for the presence of pathogens or opportunistic pathogens and to estimate the numbers of these and other organisms present in a given weight (usually 1 g) or volume (usually 100 ml).

Sampling

Solid samples should be collected in plastic jars or bags. Glass containers are undesirable, especially in food-handling premises, as they may be broken, and shards may contaminate a product. It is usual to take several samples, each of about 100 g, from different batches and/or at different times. Samples may be taken from bulk materials with spoons or scoops, previously sterilised, either in the laboratory or in boiling water for 5–10 minutes. If plastic bags are used, a bag should be turned inside out and placed over a hand, as a glove. A handful of the gloved material is then grasped and the bag everted so that the sample is now inside. Bags should be either self-sealing, or closed with Quik-Ties.

Samples of liquids, each about 100 ml, should be collected in plastic jars. A previously sterilized dipper or ladle may be used to transfer samples of bulk liquids. It is good practice to use dip slides at the same time.

Detection of pathogens

In the laboratory solid samples are homogenized mechanically and doubling dilutions made in sterile saline for culture, or tested by one of the newer 'kits', e.g for salmonellas and bacterial or fungal toxins.

It may be difficult, in some circumstances, to detect particular pathogens because they may be present in very small numbers. It is often easier to detect 'indicator organisms' which provide evidence of contamination. For example, although enteric pathogens may be present in small and undetectable numbers in a sample, they are usually accompanied by large numbers of coliform bacilli which are easily detected on suitable culture media. The presence of these 'indicates' contamination.

Counting bacteria and fungi

'Total counts'

These are done by microscopical examination of slides on which known small volumes of the material are spread, and which are then dried and stained to reveal the organisms. This method does not distinguish between living and dead organisms and the results are therefore unreliable. A newer method, the Direct Epi-Fluorescence Technique (DEFT), is more reliable. It uses stains that fluoresce only if the organisms are viable. Where possible, the diluted and homogenized sample is filtered through membranes which retain the micro-organisms. The membranes are then treated with the stain and organisms which fluoresce are counted under the microscope.

Instrumental ('automated') methods are now widely used. In some of these the sample passes through a fine orifice and an electric field which detects particles. Changes in the field, and therefore the number of particles passed, are recorded. In this method, though, some particles other than micro-organisms may be counted.

More modern instruments detect adenosine triphosphate (ATP) which is present in living organisms. The strength of the signal from ATP gives an indication of the numbers of micro-organisms.

These methods give rapid results, but cannot always be used. Alternatively, the organisms are cultured and the colonies counted, which, unfortunately, is time consuming (taking 24–48 hours).

Colony counts

Unfortunately micro-organisms usually occur in clumps containing a few to several thousand cells. Laboratories therefore report 'viable unit counts' which reflect only the numbers of organisms or clumps of organisms (units) that are able to grow under the conditions of the tests.

These manual methods of doing viable counts involve making serial tenfold dilutions of the homogenized material. Known volumes of each, usually 1 ml, are placed in petri dishes and mixed with melted culture media. Non-selective media are used to estimate the total numbers of viable units, and selective media to obtain viable counts of particular groups of organisms such as coliforms and fungi. When the media have set the dishes are incubated and colonies are counted. From these figures the number of viable units per gram may be calculated.

Alternatively, known volumes of each dilution are filtered through membranes that retain the organisms. The membranes are then placed on the surface of culture media which diffuse into them and permit the organisms to grow into countable colonies.

Dip slide counts

Dip slides (Chapter 7), originally designed for urine testing, are now widely used in industry for monitoring bacterial or fungal colony counts of liquids or suspensions. The culture media used are 'tailored' for individual processes.

Mycotoxins

Tests for mycotoxins (aflatoxins, etc.) in raw materials are specialized laboratory procedures that use 'biosensors' such as protozoa and tissue cultures (Buckle and Sanders, 1990; Robb *et al.*, 1990).

Environmental monitoring

Environmental monitoring for micro-organisms includes surveys of the microbial load of air, water and on surfaces.

Air

Air may be sampled and monitored in the workplace to determine its general microbial load and to detect airborne contamination by specific organisms from materials and arising from leakages from industrial plant. It may also be desirable to monitor air for endotoxins. Single samples are misleading and sampling should be systematic, e.g. at 2-hourly intervals at various sites. The microbial quality of the air outside the building should be measured as a baseline for comparison.

Viable counts per unit volume of air may be made by sedimentation, impaction, impinger and filtration methods. As no single culture medium will detect all kinds of micro-organisms, and some, e.g. fungi, may overgrow and obscure others, various culture media are used. These include enriched media (blood agar) for *Staphylococcus aureus*, media containing cycloheximide, which allows bacteria to grow but suppresses mould fungi, and Rose Bengal agar, which encourages fungi but suppresses bacteria. In addition, special media, designed for indicator organisms and process organisms that have escaped from industrial plant, may be used.

Sedimentation; settle plates

In this method sets of petri dishes containing various different culture media, as indicated above, are opened and left on horizontal surfaces for periods varying from 15 minutes to several hours (Figure 9.1).

They are then closed and incubated, usually at 22–30°C for saprophytes, at 37°C for pathogens and at 56°C for thermophiles. Viable micro-organisms which have settled (by gravity) on the surface of the medium will grow into colonies and can be counted. This method is useful only for assessing the numbers of larger viable units, i.e. more than 12 μm, as smaller particles settle very slowly or not at all. The results are also much affected by air currents. Settle plates are, therefore, mostly used in still air conditions in rooms, e.g in cross-contamination studies.

It is generally accepted (Gröschel, 1980) that most airborne particles of about 12 μm settle in still air at a rate of about 1 ft/min. An ordinary 4 inch diameter petri dish (ca 1/15 ft^2) will collect such viable units from 1 ft^2 of stagnant air in 15 minutes.

Impaction; slit, cascade and centrifugal samplers

These methods are useful for monitoring air in buildings and the open air, e.g. near to agricultural activities, and to detect leakages in process plants. A current of air is drawn mechanically through the instrument and impacts on the agar surface, either in petri dishes or on plastic strips.

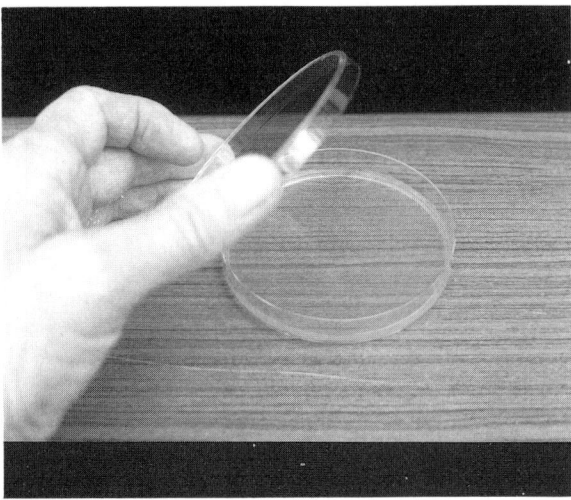

Fig. 9.1   *Settle plate.*

Slit samplers

In these instruments (Figure 9.2) a petri dish containing the culture medium is placed on a turntable in a chamber that can be closed. The turntable revolves at a predetermined rate under a narrow slit in the chamber cover, which is half the diameter of the dish in length. An electric pump draws air, usually at 700 litres/min, through the slit into the chamber and particles impact on the agar surface. The sampling time is usually 5 minutes, after which the petri dish is incubated and the number of colonies, each representing a viable unit, is counted. The total viable units of either bacteria or fungi per litre may then be calculated. Non-selective media are used for bacterial counts and selective media for counts of fungi, indicator organisms and pathogens.

Cascade samplers

These are designed to permit the numbers of particles of different sizes to be counted. They consist (Figure 9.3) of a series of four chambers, separated from each other by sieve plates which carry holes of diminishing size from the top downwards. A separate pump draws air at a pre-determined rate through the system. A petri dish of appropriate culture medium is placed in each chamber. Larger particles impact on the medium in the top chamber and progressively smaller particles impact on the agar in the lower chambers.

As with slit samplers, viable bacterial and fungal spore counts may be assessed, and pathogens and indicator organisms detected.

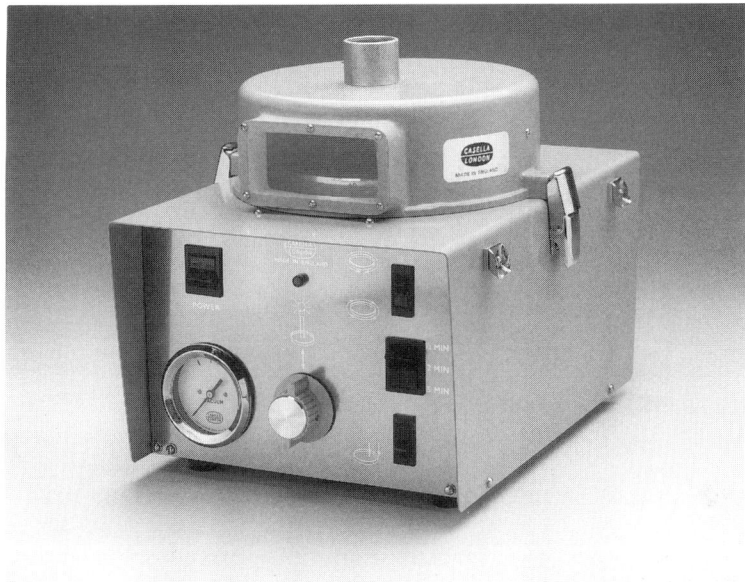

Fig. 9.2   *Slit sampler (Casella Ltd, London).*

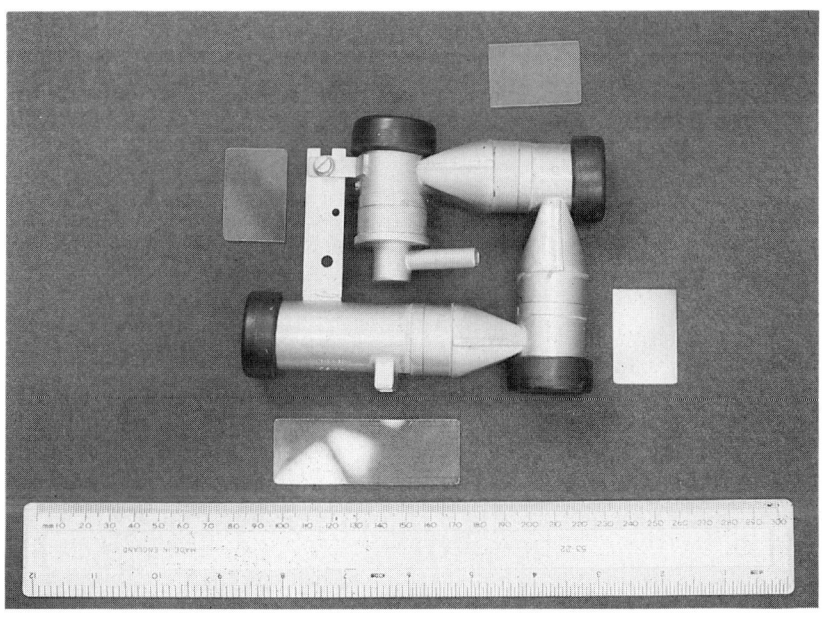

Fig. 9.3   *Cascade impactor. Courtesy of the Director, Centre for Applied Microbiology and Research, Porton.*

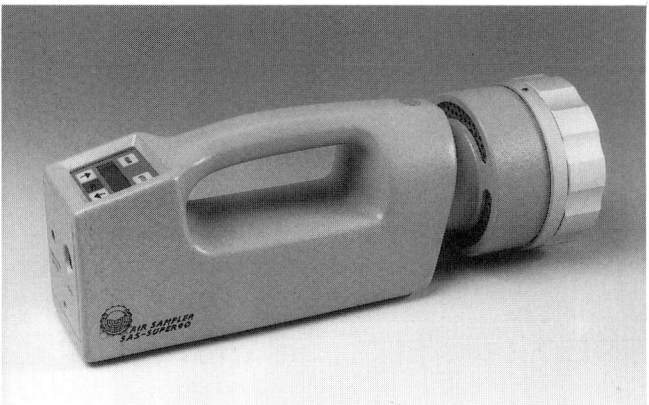

Fig. 9.4 *Biotest RCS Plus sampler—a centrifugal impactor (Biotest UK Ltd, Solihull, Birmingham).*

Impactor samplers

These samplers (Figure 9.4) are hand-held and hence more easily portable than slit or cascade samplers. In addition, they may be battery-operated as well as mains-operated. An impeller draws in air and directs it on to the surface of agar culture media.

There are two types. In the Biotest Plus Reuter Air Sampler (RCS) (Figure 9.4) the air stream is directed on to culture medium which is contained in small cells along a plastic strip. The volume of air and time of exposure of the agar is programmed by the operator. The plates or strips are incubated in the carriers provided and the number of colonies counted. The microbial load per unit volume may then be calculated.

In the Cherwell Surface Air System (SAS) the air stream is directed on to the culture medium in a petri dish (Figure 9.5).

Plates and strips containing a variety of culture media, for total viable bacterial and fungal spore counts, as well as pathogens and indicator organisms, are available.

Impinger

These are simple instruments to use, but subsequently require micro-biological expertise. They consist of glass vessels with inlet and outlet tubes (Figure 9.6) resembling chemical Drechsel bottles, from which air is extracted by a metered pump. Incoming air, collected by a sampling probe, impinges a few millimetres above the surface of a liquid culture medium.

After sampling, the vessel is returned to the laboratory where viable counts

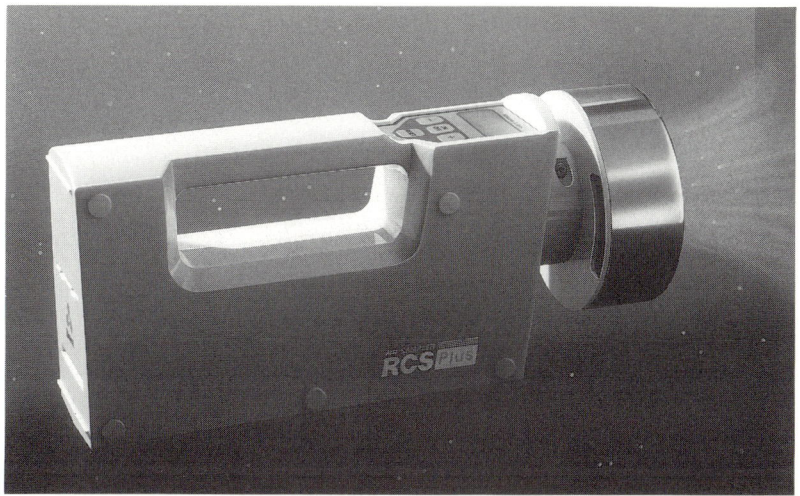

Fig. 9.5   *SAS Sampler—a sieve plate impactor (Cherwell Laboratories Ltd, Bicester, Oxon).*

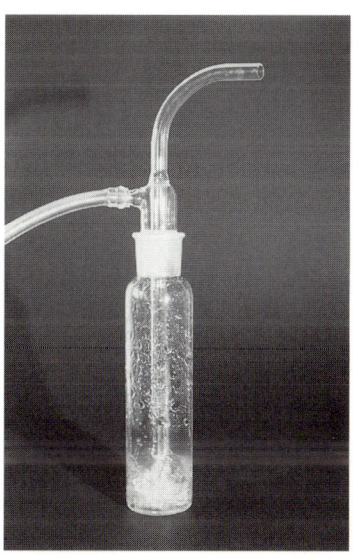

Fig. 9.6   *Glass impinger. Courtesy of the Director, Centre for Applied Microbiology and Research, Porton.*

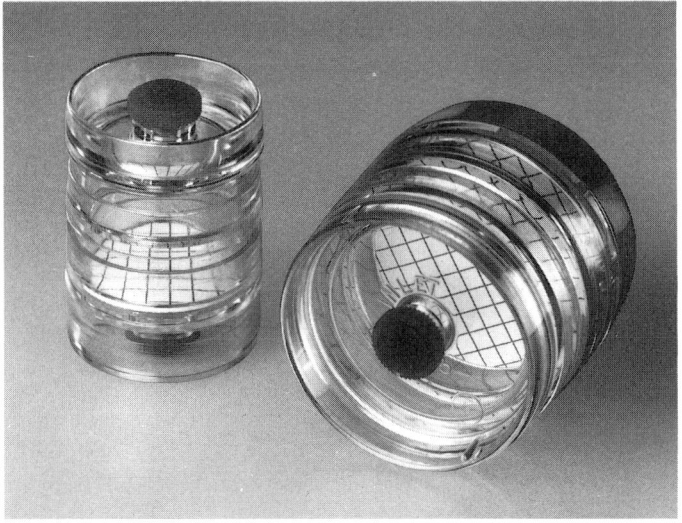

Fig. 9.7   *Membrane filter (Millipore, Watford, Herts).*

are done on the fluid by spreading measured volumes of serial dilutions on suitable culture media, incubating and counting colonies.

Filtration

There are several samplers that depend on the filtration of measured volumes of air through cellulose acetate membranes which retain the micro-organisms (Figure 9.7). The membrane is then placed on the surface of culture medium, incubated and colonies are counted. A disadvantage of these is that the air stream may dehydrate the organisms and render them non-viable. Such dehydration is avoided in a newer instrument which uses moist, gelatin membrane filters (Figure 9.8). The flow rate and time may be selected and the flexible hose permits the sampler to be placed well away from the pump.

For technical details of some of these samplers, and their relative advantages and disadvantages, see Hambleton *et al.* (1992) and Crook (1995). The manufacturers' data sheets are also useful.

Standards

There are no official standards for the microbial content of air but, in general, whatever method is used, the indoor air should not have bacterial or fungal counts of more than 200 colony-forming units per m^3 above that of the outdoor air. Particular attention should be paid to the presence of *Aspergillus*

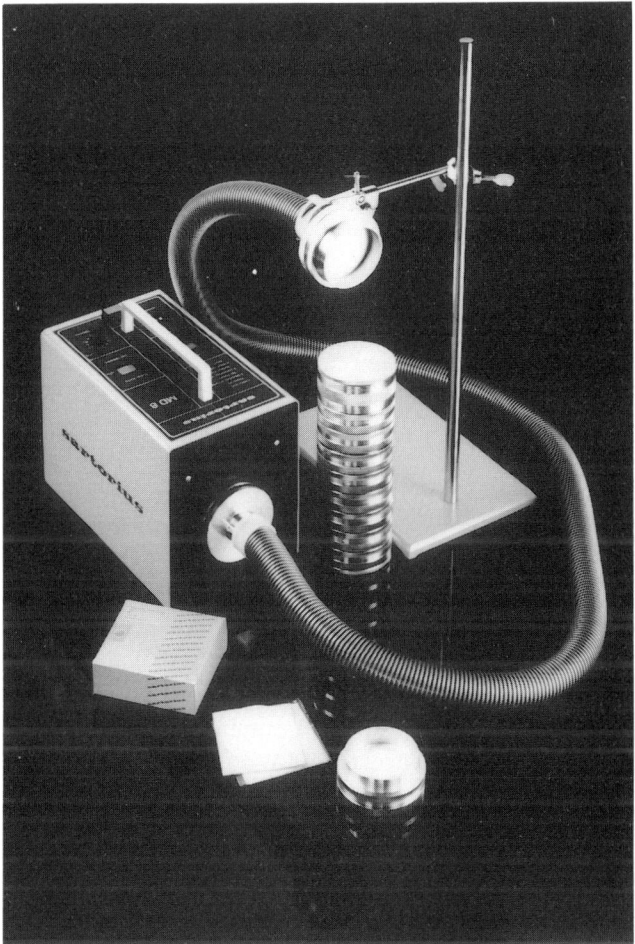

Fig. 9.8 *Gelatin membrane air sampler (Sartorius Ltd, Epsom, Surrey).*

fumigatus, Pseudomonas aeruginosa and *Staphylococcus aureus*, which will be identified by the laboratory.

Table 2.1 (p. 11) gives examples of bacterial loads in the air at various sites.

Detection of endotoxins

Airborne dust is usually examined. It is sampled by the membrane method, as above. The dust is washed from the membrane and tested with a (commercial) Limulus amoebocyte kit. Endotoxins gel the amoebocytes.

Water

In developed countries there is little point in monitoring mains water supplies. Public health and utility authorities do this regularly and frequently. Private bore hole supplies, process waters and other private waters, e.g. of bathing facilities, pleasure pools and spas, to which workers and sports enthusiasts are exposed, may require testing to ensure that they are not contaminated with micro-organisms injurious to health. This is best done by an experienced laboratory, but it is desirable that local staff are aware of what is involved.

Total viable counts on water samples are so variable as to be of little value. It is quite difficult to isolate pathogenic bacteria from water (but see legionnaires' disease, below) because, if present, they are there in only small numbers. This is why indicator organisms are sought. They are more easily detected and counted and are evidence of contamination, e.g. by sewage. The coliform bacillus, *Escherichia coli*, is the indicator organism most frequently used to monitor for faecal pollution, but there are others such as enterococci ('faecal streptococci') and clostridia.

The technique consists of passing the sample, which may be several litres, through membrane filters, similar to those mentioned above for air monitoring, except that the equipment (Figure 9.9) is more sophisticated (although single use, disposable filters are available commercially). The membranes are placed on culture media and incubated. Colonies which grow are identified by bacteriological techniques.

There are agreed standards for the presence/absence of coliform bacteria

Table 9.1   *Drinking water standards*

	Maximum admissible concentrations
Parameter:	
Total coliforms	None detected in 100 ml sample
Faecal coliforms	None detected in 100 ml sample
Faecal streptococci	None detected in 100 ml sample
Sulphite-reducing clostrida	Not more than 1 in 20 ml sample
Guideline:	
Total viable count	at 37°C, 10 in 1 ml at 22°C, 100 in 1 ml

For treated water the values should be considerably lower at the point where it leaves the processing plant.
From: EC Directive 80/78/EEC (European Commission, 1980).

Table 9.2   *European Union bacteriological guide levels for bathing waters (figures are viable counts per 100 ml of water)*

	Excellent	Satisfactory	Poor
Total coliforms	≤ 500	500–10 000	>10 000
Faecal coli	≤ 100	100–2 000	>2 000
Faecal streptococci	≤ 100	100–2 000	>2 000

From EC Directive 76/160 EEC (European Commission, 1976).

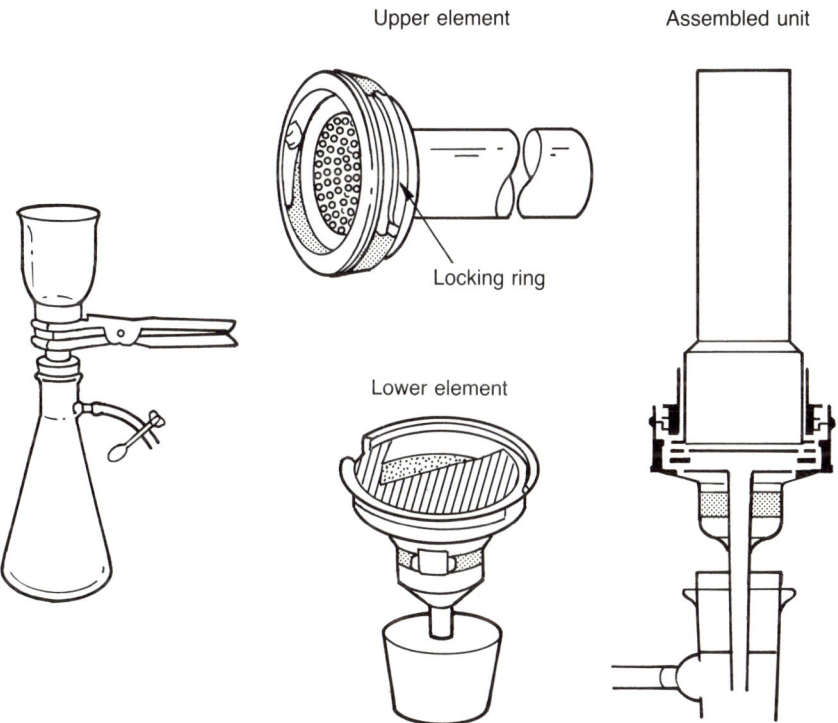

Fig. 9.9   *Membrane filter apparatus for water sampling. Reproduced from* Medical Laboratory Manual for Tropical Countries *vol. 1 (Butterworth-Heinemann, Oxford), courtesy of Miss Monica Cheesbrough and Dr B. Lloyd.*

and other micro-organisms in drinking waters (Table 9.1) and recreational waters (Table 9.2).

There are exceptions to the policy of seeking indicator organisms rather than pathogens. These include investigations into outbreaks of legionnaires' disease, and the monitoring of cooling towers and air-conditioning plants for

Legionella pneumophila, the detection in swimming pools and spas of *Staphylococcus aureus* and *Pseudomonas aeruginosa*, both of which are associated with skin and ear infections, and of leptospiras and cryptosporidia in waters used for sport and recreation. The methods involved require a great deal of microbiological expertise and frequently very large volumes of suspect waters have to be tested. It is essential that the laboratory be consulted.

Surfaces

The assessment of microbial contamination and the detection of pathogens on surfaces are important aspects of environmental monitoring. The simplest and most practical procedures are the swab technique and the contact plate. Both methods permit counts to be made of micro-organisms on surfaces, and organisms that grow may be identified by microbiological methods. There are also instrumental methods.

The swab method

This may be used on flat or curved surfaces and on entire objects or sample areas. A sterile swab, which is cotton wool wrapped tightly on a wooden stick or a wire (Figure 7.1a, p. 100), and contained in glass or plastic tube, is moistened with sterile culture medium or saline and rubbed over the surface to be sampled. It is then replaced in its tube and sent to the laboratory where it is used to inoculate culture media for colony counting. For sampling specific areas a template is made of card by cutting out an area of, e.g. 100 cm^2. This is placed on the surface to be tested and the swab is rubbed over the exposed area.

The contact method

There are two methods. One uses a flexible plastic carrier containing the culture medium and can be applied to surfaces that are not flat (Figure 9.10a). After application to the surface it is returned to its container and incubated. The other employs small, shallow petri dishes (Figure 9.10b), the bottom parts of which are filled to the brim with culture media so that a slightly convex surface is exposed. The lid is removed, the plate is pressed firmly on the test surface and then removed, covered and incubated. Colonies are then counted.

Instrumental method

The adenosine triphosphate method, mentioned above and which gives more immediate results, has also been adapted for assessing microbial contamination of surfaces, and instruments are available commercially.

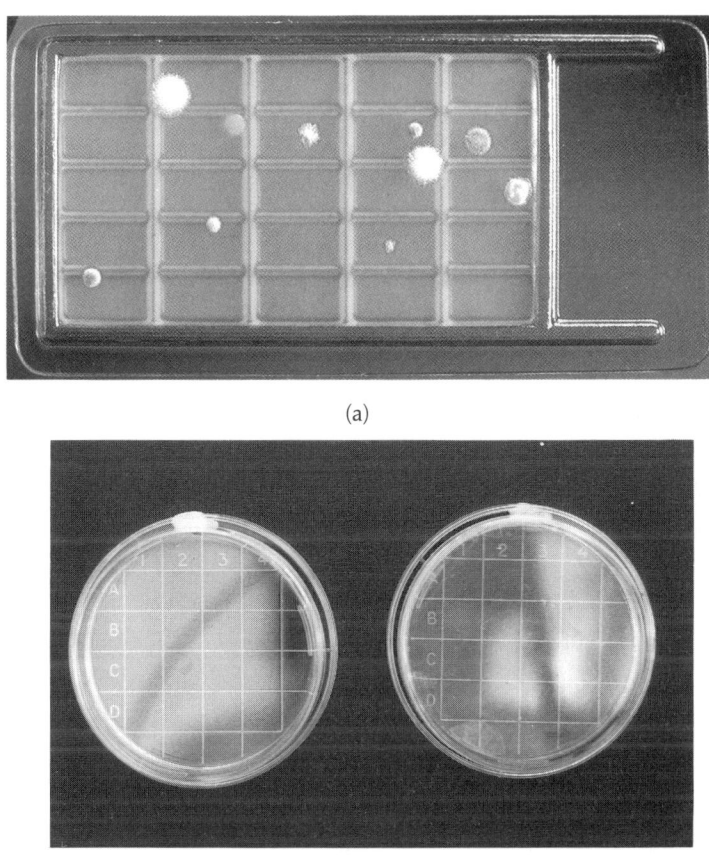

(a)

(b)

Fig. 9.10 *Contact plates for surface sampling: (a) plastic, for curved surfaces (Biotest UK Ltd, Solihull, Birmingham); (b) replica plate for flat surfaces.*

Detection of blood

Small splashes and droplets of blood may not be visible to the naked eye but still contain large numbers of infectious particles, e.g. the hepatitis B virus. The following method, derived from that of Beaumont (1987), uses a proprietary product, Haemostix (Ames Co., Miles Laboratories, Stoke Poges, Slough), employed in hospitals and clinics for detecting blood in urine. Cotton-wool throat swabs (Figure 7.1a, p. 100), and small (e.g. 25 ml) screw-capped bottles containing 1 ml of sterile saline are also required. A swab is removed from its tube, dipped in the saline and then rubbed over the surface to be examined. It is then placed in the screw-capped bottle and the stick is broken off so that the bottle, containing only the swab, may be capped. The contents of the bottle are then mixed well, preferably with a laboratory vortex mixer, for 10–15 minutes. A Haemostix is then dipped into the fluid, removed, drained and any colour change observed. A change from yellow to green or dark blue indicates the presence of blood. The method is very sensitive and will detect blood diluted $1:10^4$ in saline.

Further information

For further information about: (1) sampling air, see Crook and Lacey (1988); Ashton and Gill (1992); Collins (1993); (2) sampling water and surfaces, see Collins and Grange (1990); Collins *et al.* (1995); (3) sampling biotechnological processes, see Hambleton *et al.* (1992); Tuijnenberg-Muijs (1992); and (4) laboratory procedures, see Collins *et al.* (1995).

10 Legal protection and official advice

Microbial diseases prescribed for industrial injuries benefit and those for which notification is required to safeguard the health of the community are considered in Chapter 1. Other legislation concerned with protection against microbial diseases—infections and allergies—is considered here.

Before 1974 the only pieces of legislation designed to protect industrial workers from an infectious agent were the various anthrax orders and regulations. Several official and independent UK publications on the prevention of infection in laboratories appeared both before and after the *Health and Safety at Work etc. Act, 1974* (Collins *et al.*, 1974; UK Health Departments, 1978; HSE, 1991b, Collins, 1983, 1993) but these were largely advisory and served only as guidance until recently.

The Health and Safety at Work etc. Act 1974 (HSAWA)

This is the primary UK legislation that is intended to protect the health and safety of workers (and others). In general, it lays legal obligations on employers and employees to provide a 'safe system of work', i.e. a working environment and working practices, that does not place any person, whether employed or not, at risk of injury or disease. It is an 'enabling' act under which various regulations are made. The Health and Safety Commission (HSC) was created under this act. The Health and Safety Executive (HSE) is the Commission's executive body and embraces the various factory and other inspectorates.

The medical arm of HSE is the Employment Medical Advisory Service (EMAS) (see Chapter 7), which, among other things, gives advice to government bodies, general medical practitioners, industry and the public on matters relating to health at work. The HSC and HSE are also served by several advisory committees. Those concerned with microbial disease, mainly laboratory or hospital associated, are the Advisory Committee on Dangerous Pathogens (ACDP), and various Health Service advisory committees. The Advisory Committee on Genetic Manipulation (ACGM) gives advice on the contained use and controlled release of genetically modified organisms.

The Reporting of Injuries, Diseases and Dangerous Occurrences Regulations 1995 (RIDDOR)

These regulations, outlined in Chapter 1 of this book, replaced some existing regulations concerning the reporting of industrial diseases under the old Factories Act with new requirements for reporting job-associated diseases, etc. Accidents may not cause injuries at the time, but are classed as dangerous occurrences if there is a potential for subsequent injury or infection. Reportable occupational infections and allergies are listed in Table 1.4 (p. 6). Laboratory-acquired infections, even if not listed, are also included.

Microbial diseases that occur in factories and on farms must be reported to the HSE; those occurring in offices, shops and restaurants to the local Environmental Health Department.

The Control of Substances Hazardous to Health Regulations 1994 (COSHH)

These regulations, originally introduced in 1988, were designed to protect workers from any hazardous substances that they might encounter during their normal occupations. These regulations now embody the EC *Directive on the Protection of Workers from the Risks Related to Exposure to Biological Agents at Work* (European Commission, 1990) (known as 'The Biological Agents Directive'). They place duties on both employers and employees.

Employers are required to:

- identify hazardous substances;
- assess the risks involved in handling those substances, particularly in respect of the ways in which they may enter or affect the human body (see Chapter 3), and then make informed judgements about actions necessary to remove or reduce these risks;
- provide workers with information about hazardous substances;
- train workers in the handling of hazardous substances;
- introduce such control measures as are reasonable, e.g:
  —remove the hazardous substances, or replace them by those that are less hazardous;
  —reduce the level of exposure;
  —isolate the area where they are handled;
  —identify people at risk;
  —minimize the number of people at risk;
  —test and monitor these control measures;
  —monitor and record exposures to hazardous substances;

—arrange health surveillance programmes;
—supply protective equipment.

Employees have duties to:

- accept training;
- use safe methods;
- use protective equipment;
- use control measures properly;
- read and understand labels on materials and substances;
- report hazards;
- accept health surveillance.

Most of these requirements will already be in place, under the 1988 COSHH regulations. The assessment of risks in work with micro-organisms, required in the 1994 regulations, however, introduces a new dimension.

COSHH and work with micro-organisms

Although the 1988 COSHH regulations included micro-organisms as biological substances, there was little information or direction on assessing the risks of handling them under industrial conditions.

For laboratory workers, however, as indicated above, there was some guidance, in the form of a classification of micro-organisms on the basis of hazard into four Hazard Groups, ranging from those (Group 1) that are unlikely to cause human disease to those (Group 4) that may cause very serious disease. Such a scheme was introduced in the USA by the Centers for Disease Control in 1969–1974 (CDC, 1974), later adopted by the World Health Organization (1979, 1993) and in the UK, by the Advisory Committee on Dangerous Pathogens (HSE, 1984, 1990b, 1995a) (see below). This system permitted the formulation of sets of precautions, 'Containment' (or 'Biosafety') levels for each group that included technical methods, building construction, equipment and processes. The system was originally drawn up in respect of laboratory-acquired infections but was adapted to industry by the Organization for Economic Cooperation and Development (OECD, 1986) and the European Federation of Biotechnology (Frommer *et al.* 1992).

When the European Union's *Directive on the Protection of Workers from Risks Related to Exposure to Biological Agents at Work* (European Commission, 1990) was incorporated in the 1994 COSHH regulations the Hazard Group classification was retained but the term 'biological agent' is used instead of 'pathogen'. This classification system is shown in Table 10.1, but as it relates only to infections, any organisms in Group 1, which may be responsible for other disease such as allergies, are included and require risk assessments.

Table 10.1   *Classification of micro-organisms into groups on the basis of hazard*

Group 1	Agents that are most unlikely to cause human disease.
Group 2	Agents that can cause human disease and might be a hazard to workers; they are unlikely to spread in the community; effective prophylaxis and/or treatment are usually available.
Group 3	Agents that can cause severe human disease and which present a serious hazard to workers; there may be a risk of spread in the community; effective prophylaxis and/or treatment are usually available.
Group 4	Agents that cause severe human disease and present a serious hazard to workers; there may be a high risk of spread in the community; effective prophylaxis and treatment are not available.

Adapted from *The Control of Substances Hazardous to Health Regulations 1994* (HSE, 1994b). Crown copyright is reproduced with the permission of the Controller of HMSO.

The 1994 COSHH regulations extend those of 1988 to include in detail the risks arising from exposure to micro-organisms and other biological agents and include an appropriate code of practice in addition to that which accompanied the 1988 regulations. A distinction is drawn between activities in which there is a deliberate intention to work with an agent, and activities where exposure is incidental, e.g. in agriculture, refuse handling and healthcare.

According to the regulations a biological agent is '. . . any micro-organism, cell culture or human endoparasite, including any which have been genetically modified, which may cause any infection, allergy, toxicity, or otherwise create a hazard to human health'.

An 'approved classification' is provided, listing agents in Hazard Groups 2, 3 and 4. This may be amended from time to time. The current list is given in a UK publication (HSE, 1995a). Table 10.2 lists the organisms mentioned in this book and the Hazard Groups into which they have been placed.

The new regulations absorb and replace the notification requirements of the *Health and Safety (Dangerous Pathogens) Regulations, 1981*. They require, among other things:

- keeping lists of exposed workers where there is the deliberate use of agents in Hazard Groups 3 and 4;
- keeping as low as possible the numbers of employees exposed, or likely to be exposed, to biological agents;
- designing processes and control measures that avoid or minimize release of agents into the environment;

Table 10.2 *Hazard groups of micro-organisms mentioned in this book**

Organisms	Hazard group	Organisms	Hazard group
Acanthamoeba spp.	2	Kyasanur Forest virus	4
Acinetobacter spp.	2	Lassa fever virus	4
Alkaligenes spp.	2	*Legionella pneumophila*	2
Ankylostoma duodenale	2	*Leishmania donovani*	3
Ascaris lumbricoides	2	*Leishmania braziliensis*	3
Aspergillus fumigatus	2	*Leptospira interrogans*	2
Astroviruses	2	*Listeria monocytogenes*	2
Bacillus anthracis	3	Louping ill virus	3
Bacillus cereus	2	Lymphocytic choriomeningitis	
Bordetella pertussis	2	virus	3
Borrelia burgdorferi	2	Marburg virus	4
Borrelia duttoni	2	Measles virus	2
Borrelia recurrentis	2	*Microsporon* spp.	2
Brucella spp.	3	*Moraxella* spp.	2
Campylobacter jejuni	2	*Morganella* spp.	2
Chlamydia psittaci	3	Mumps virus	2
Clostridium spp.	2	*Mycobacterium bovis*	3
Corynebacterium diphtheriae	2	*Mycobacterium chelonei*	2
Coxiella burnetii	2	*Mycobacterium marinum*	2
Creutzfeldt–Jakob agent	4	*Mycobacterium fortuitum*	2
Cryptosporidium spp.	2	*Myocabacterium terrae*	2
Cytomegalovirus	2	*Mycobacterium tuberculosis*	3
Ebola virus	4	*Mycoplasma* spp.	2
Echinococcus granulosum	3	*Naegleria fowleri*	3
Entamoeba histolytica	2	*Neisseria meningitidis*	2
Enterobacter spp.	2	Newcastle disease virus	2
Enterobius vermicularis	2	*Nocardia* spp.	2
Erysipelothrix rhusiopathiae	2	Orf virus	2
Escherichia coli	2	Paravaccinia virus	2
Francisella tularensis	3	Parvovirus	2
Giardia lamblia	2	*Pasteurella multocida*	2
Hantaviruses	3	*Plasmodium falciparum*	3
Helicobacter pylori	2	*Plasmodium*, other spp.	2
Hepatitis A virus	2	Poliovirus	2
Hepatitis B, C and E viruses	3	*Proteus* spp.	2
Herpes simplex virus	2	*Pseudomonas mallei*	3
Human immunodeficiency virus	3	Rabies virus	3
Influenza virus	2	Respiratory syncytial virus	2
Klebsiella spp.	2	*Rickettsia* spp.	3

(*continued*)

Table 10.2 (*continued*)

Organisms	Hazard group	Organisms	Hazard group
Rochalimaea spp.	2	*Taenia saginata*	2
Rotavirus	2	*Toxocara canis*	2
Rubella virus	2	*Toxocara cati*	2
Salmonella typhi	3	*Toxoplasma gondii*	2
Salmonella, other spp.	2	*Treponema pallidum*	2
Schistosoma spp.	2	*Trichophyton* spp.	2
Serratia marcescens	2	*Trypanosoma brucei*	3
Shigella sonnei	2	*Trypanosoma rhodesiense*	3
Shigella flexneri	2	*Trypanosoma cruzi*	3
Simian B virus	4	'Unconventional agents'†	3
Spirillum minus	2	Varicella zoster virus	2
Sporotrichum schenckii	2	Vesicular stomatitis virus	2
Streptobacillus moniliformis	2	*Vibrio cholerae*	2
Staphylococcus aureus	2	*Vibrio parahaemolyticus*	2
Streptococcus suis	2	*Yersinia pestis*	3
Streptococcus, other spp.	2		

* According to the Dangerous Pathogens Advisory Group (HSE, 1994a, 1995a). Organisms not listed are assumed to be in Group 1.

† Agents of transmissible spongiform encephalopathies.

- display of Biohazard signs where appropriate;
- notification to a competent authority (HSE) of certain activities involving biological agents;
- notification to HSE of intention to use, for the first time, agents in Hazard Groups 2, 3 and 4;
- employees to be given written information about serious accident procedures, the handling of the most hazardous agents, and the reporting of accidents and incidents;
- provision of appropriate protective clothing and equipment;
- prevention of the transmission of biological agents by protective equipment;
- keeping medical, exposure and vaccination records;
- notification to HSE of intended consignment.

The HSE publishes a number of leaflets that give guidance to workers and employers on various aspects of diseases caused by biological agents. These are listed in Appendix 2.

Assessment of risk

Unlike chemicals, where hazard data are available from manufacturers and tables giving maximum exposure limits (MELs) and threshold limit values (TLVs) are published by the HSE and are revised annually (HSE 1995b), no such information is available for infectious doses of micro-organisms. There are many uncertainties in work with these biological agents, e.g. the numbers present, their place of origin and the virulence of a given strain. Assessments are therefore more difficult than those relating to chemicals. One may begin with a classification system of which recognizes three categories of exposure:

Category 1. Frequent occupational exposure.
Category 2. Possible occupational exposure.
Category 3. No exposure.

The risk assessment in respect of employees in Category 1 should be strict and detailed. For those in Category 2 it may be less strict and detailed, while no assessment is necessary for employees in Category 3.

The following questions will assist in making an assessment.

- which agents are to be used and in which Hazard Group(s) are they?
- what other agents might be present, e.g as microbial contaminants, tumour agents in cell cultures, hazardous proteins, unidentified agents such as those of transmissible spongiform encephalopathies?
- in what form are these agents—viruses, vegetative bacteria, spores?
- how resistant are they to chemical and physical agents?
- how are they transmitted—airborne, by ingestion or injection, by vectors?
- how serious is the disease they may cause?
- what is the likelihood of exposure and of subsequent disease?
- how many workers might be exposed, how much and for how long?
- are any workers particularly susceptible?
- is there any previous experience of the results of exposure?

Answers to these questions should indicate the appropriate physical and medical control measures.

Control measures

The COSHH regulations and codes of practice give clear guidance.

Appropriate containment measures for laboratory work are shown in Table 10.3, and for industry in Table 10.4.

Table 10.3   *Summary of containment levels for laboratory use of micro-organisms in Hazard Groups 1, 2, and 3**

Requirement	Containment level		
	1	2	3
Isolation of laboratory	No	No	Yes
Room sealable for decontamination	No	No	Yes
Ventilation:			
inward air flow	No	Op	Yes
mechanical via building system	No	Op	Op
mechanical, independent	No	No	Yes
filtered air exhaust	No	No	Yes
Effluent treatment	No	No	No
Autoclave:			
on site	Yes	Yes	Yes
in laboratory room	No	No	Yes
double-ended	No	No	Op
Microbiological safety cabinet:			
Class I or II	No	Yes	Yes
Class III	No	No	Op

* Containment Level 4 is omitted because very few laboratories handle agents in Hazard Group 4.
Op = optional.
Adapted from HSE (1990b). Crown copyright is reproduced with the permission of the Controller of HMSO.

For laboratories and industries that use micro-organisms further guidance is available: (1) in medical diagnosis and research, HSE (1990b, 1991b); Collins (1993); WHO (1993); (2) in industry and other workplaces, Küenzi *et al.* (1985, 1987); Frommer *et al.* (1989, 1992, 1993); Collins and Grange (1990); Collins and Beale (1992); OECD, 1992: Lelieveld *et al.* (1995).

The World Health Organization (WHO, 1995) has produced guidelines on the production of vaccines and biological products.

Genetically modified organisms (GMOs)

Although the WHO (1982a), the European Federation of Biotechnology (Küenzi *et al.*, 1985; Frommer *et al.*, 1989, Lieberman *et al.*, 1991), the

Table 10.4   *Summary of containment measures for the industrial use of micro-organisms in Hazard Groups 2 and 3**

Measures	Level 2	Level 3
Closed systems	Yes	Yes
Exhaust gases	Minimize release	Prevent release
Sample collection	Minimize release	Prevent release
	Validated method	Validated chemical or physical methods
Inactivation of bulk culture fluids	Minimize release	Prevent release
Equipment seals	Optional	Optional
Closed systems within controlled area	Optional	Yes
Biohazard signs	Optional	Yes
Restricted access	Yes	Yes
Protective clothing	No	Yes
Shower on leaving controlled area	No	Optional
Sink effluents treated before disposal	No	Optional
Adequate ventilation of controlled area	Optional	Optional
Controlled area at negative air pressure	No	Optional
Input/extract air HEPA filtered	No	Optional
Spillage contained within controlled area	Optional	Yes
Controlled area sealable for fumigation	Optional	Yes
Process effluent treated before disposal	Inactivated by validated means	Inactivated by validated chemical or physical methods

* Hazard Group 1 micro-organisms are handled under Good Industrial Large Scale Practice (GILSP).
Adapted from HSE (1995a). Crown copyright is reproduced with the permission of the Controller of HMSO.

Organization for Economic Cooperation and Development (OECD, 1992) do not consider that genetically modified organisms (GMOs) offer any greater risks than those that occur naturally, and that measures to contain the latter are fully effective for the former, GMOs are given special legal status in respect of contained use and deliberate release by *The Genetically Modified Organisms (Contained Use) Regulations 1992*, which implement the European Commission (1990a) Directive 90/219/EEC, and *The Genetically Modified*

Organisms (Deliberate Release) Regulations 1992, which implement the European Commission (1990b) Directive 90/220/EEC. (Further revision of this is expected.)

These regulations recognize two groups of GMOs: in general Group I includes those where 'The recipient or parental micro-organism is unlikely to cause disease to humans, animals or plants'; and those in Group II where 'The nature of the vector and the insert is such that they do not endow the genetically-modified organism with a phenotype likely to cause disease in humans, animals or plants, or to cause adverse effects in the environment'. The GMO containment regulations are more stringent than those for naturally occurring micro-organisms and compliance with GMO regulations satisfies those for COSHH. Problems may arise when an organism normally in Hazard Group 1 falls into GMO Group II because of (a) environmental risks, even though it is unlikely to cause human disease, or (b) is derived by genetic modification from a pathogen. In the latter case containment measures may be appropriate to reduced virulence. If there is a mismatch the more stringent regulations apply.

Other legislation

There is very little other legislation pertaining to the use of, or work involving contact with, micro-organisms. The titles of the relevant acts, orders and regulations are listed in Appendix 1.

Appendix 1

Relevant UK legislation

The Anthrax Prevention Order 1971
The Anthrax Prevention Order (Exemptions) Regulations 1981
The Health and Safety at Work etc. Act 1974
The Public Health (Control of Diseases) Act 1984
The Social Security (Industrial Diseases)(Prescribed Diseases) Regulations 1995
The Reporting of Injuries, Diseases and Dangerous Occurrences Regulations 1985
The Management of the Health and Safety at Work Regulations 1992
The Genetically Modified Organisms (Contained Use) Regulations 1992
The Genetically Modified Organisms (Deliberate Release) Regulations 1992
The Notification of Cooling Towers and Evaporative Condensers Regulations 1992
The Control of Substances Hazardous to Health Regulations 1994

These may be obtained from Her Majesty's Stationery Office.

Appendix 2

Some relevant leaflets, etc. issued at no cost by the Health and Safety Executive

INDG 136L	*COSHH. A brief guide for employers*
HSE 31	*RIDDOR. Everyone's guide to RIDDOR 95*
IACL 25A	*Agriculture: health carry card*
AS5	*Farmer's lung*
INDG 84	*Leptospirosis*
INDG 85	*Bovine spongiform encephalopathy (BSE)*
INDG 140L	*Grain dust leaflet*
SIR 34	*Occupational exposure to grain dust*
NIS/09/03	*Grain dust—maximum exposure limit*
IACL 28	*Humidifier fever in the print industry*
INDG 167L	*Health risks from metal-working fluids*
INDG 168L	*Metal-working fluids: a guide to good practice*
INDG 169L	*Cutting fluids and you*
MS(B) 12	*Save your breath. Campaign against occupational lung disease—advice for employees*
MS(B) 16	*Save your breath. Campaign against occupational lung disease. A guide for employers*
INDG 95L	*Breathe Freely. Respiratory sensitizers and COSHH—on preventing occupational asthma*
IAC L27	*Legionnaires' disease*
NIS/18/01	*Needlestick injuries (HSE Information sheet)*
INDG 198L	*Working with sewage. The health hazards*
INDG 197L	*Working with sewage: health carry card*
—	*Agriculture Information Sheet No. 2. Zoonoses in agriculture. Preventing the spread of disease in livestock handlers*
—	*Staying healthy. A guide for workers in farming, forestry and horticulure*

These may be obtained from HSE Books, PO Box 1999, Sudbury, Suffolk CO10 6FS.

Appendix 3

Useful addresses

The Amateur Rowing Association, 6 Lower Mall, London W6. Tel. 0181 741 5314.

British Occupational Hygiene Society (BOHS), Suite 2, Georgian House, Great Northern Road, Derby DE1 1LT. Tel. 01332 298101.

Communicable Diseases Surveillance Centre, 61 Colindale Avenue, London NW9 5EQ. Tel. 0181 200 6868.

Department of Environmental and Occupational Medicine, University of Aberdeen, University Medical School, Foresterhill, Aberdeen AB9 2ZD. Tel. 01224 681818.

Department of Occupational Health, University of Manchester, Stopford Building, Oxford Road, Manchester M13 9PT. Tel. 0161 275 5522.

Faculty of Occupational Medicine, The Royal College of Physicians, 6 St Andrew's Place, Regent's Park, London NW1 4LB. Tel. 0171 487 3414.

Health Education Authority, Hamilton House, Mabledon Place, London WC1H 9TX. Tel 0171 383 3833.

Health and Safety Executive, Rose Court, Southwark Bridge Road, London SE1 9HS. Tel. 0171 717 6000 (for local offices see telephone directory).

HSE Books, Library and Information Service, Broad Lane, Sheffield S3 7HQ. Tel. 0114 289 2000.

HSE Books, Mail Order, PO Box 1999, Sudbury, Suffolk CO10 6FS. Tel. 01787 881165.

Institute of Occupational Health (Birmingham), The University of Birmingham, Edgbaston, Birmingham B15 2TT. Tel. 0121 414 3344.

Institute of Occupational Hygienists, Suite 2, Georgian House, Great Northern Road, Derby DE1 1LT. Tel. 0133 298087.

Institute of Occupational Medicine (Edinburgh), 8 Roxburgh Place, Edinburgh EH8 9SE. Tel. 0131 667 5131.

Institute of Occupational Safety and Health (IOSH), The Grange, Highfield Drive, Wigston, Leicester LE18 1NN. Tel. 0116 257 1399.

London School of Hygiene and Tropical Medicine, Keppel Street, London WC1N 7HT. Tel. 0171 636 8636.

Scottish Sports Council, Caledonia House, Southgyle, Edinburgh EH12 9DQ. Tel. 0131 317 7200.

Society of Occupational Health Nursing, Royal College of Nursing, 20 Cavendish Square, London W1M 0AB. Tel. 0171 409 3333.

Society of Occupational Medicine, 6 St Andrew's Place, Regent's Park, London NW1 4LB. Tel. 0171 486 2641.

Sports Council of Wales, National Sports Centre, Cardiff CF1 9SW. Tel. 01222 397571.

Universities Occupational Health Service, 10 Parks Road, Oxford OX1 3PD. Tel. 01865 282676.

Wolfson Institute (Dundee), c/o Ninewells Hospital, Dundee DE1 9SY. Tel. 01382 660111.

References

Acha, P.N. and Szyfres, B. (1989) *Zoonoses and Communicable Diseases Common to Man and Animals*, 2nd edn, Washington, Pan American Health Organization

Agar, B.P. and Tickner, J.A. (1985) *The Control of Microorganisms responsible for Legionnaires' Disease and Humidifier Fever, Occupational Hygiene Monograph No. 14*, Leeds, Science Reviews

Agrup, G., Belin, L., Sjöstedt, L. and Skerfving, S. (1986) Allergy to laboratory animals among laboratory technicians and animal keepers. *Br. J. Ind. Med.* **43**, 192–198

Allsop, D. and Seal, K.J. (1986) *Introduction to Biodeterioration*, London, Edward Arnold, pp. 34–39

Alter, M.J. (1993) The detection, transmission and outcome of hepatitis C virus infection. *Inf. Agents Dis.*, **2**, 155–166

Angus, K.N. (1983) Cryptosporidiosis in man, domestic animals and birds; a review. *J. Roy. Soc. Med.*, **76**, 62–70

Ancona, A. (1990) *Occupational Skin Disease* 2nd edn (ed. R.M. Adams,), Philadelphia, Saunders, pp. 89–112

Anon. (1981) Shipyard eye. *Br. Med. J.*, **283**, 629–630

Anon. (1987) Poultry workers. *Bull. Inst. Occup. Hlth*, Winter 1987, No. 4, p. 2

Anon. (1988) Nosocomial legionella outbreak due to shower mist inhalation. *Hosp. Infect. Control*, **16**, 67–68

Anon. (1990) Hantaviruses (Editorial). *Lancet*, **336**, 407–408

Ashton, I.A. and Gill, F.S. (1992) *Monitoring for Health Hazards in the Environment*, 2nd edn, Oxford, Blackwell, pp. 189–217

Astbury, C.V. and Baxter, P.J. (1990) Infection risks in hospital staff from blood: hazardous injury rates and acceptance of hepatitis B immunisation. *J. Soc. Occ. Med*, **40**, 92–93

Australian National University (1990) *Health in the Tropics. A survival guide for travellers and field workers*, Canberra, Australia

Bartlett, C.R.L., Macrae, A.D. and Macfarlane, J.T. (1986) *Legionella Infections*, London, Edward Arnold, 156pp

Basel Forum on Biosafety (1993) *Biosafety of Mammalian Cell Cultures*, (Swiss) Basel, Agency for Biosafety Research and Assessment of Technology Impact

Beale, A.J. (1992) Safe handling of mammalian cells on an industrial scale. In *Safety in Industrial Microbiology and Biotechnology* (eds C.H. Collins and A.J. Beale). Oxford, Butterworth-Heinemann, pp. 153–160

Beaumont, L.R. (1987) The detection of blood on nonporous surfaces. *Inf. Control*, **8**, 424–426

Beck-Sague, C., Jarvis, W.R., Fruehling, J.R., *et al.* (1991) Universal precautions and mortuary practitioners: influences on practice and risk of occupationally acquired infection. *J. Occup. Med.*, **33**, 874–878

Bell, J.C., Palmer, S.R. and Payne, J.M. (1988) *The Zoonoses. Infections transmitted from animals to man*, London, Edward Arnold

Bennett, A.M. (1987) Sensitising issues. *Lab. Pract.,* **41,** 9–12

Bennett, A.M. and Norris, K.D. (1989) *State of the Art Report No. 2. Industrial Biosafety Project,* Stevenage, Warren Springs Laboratory, pp. 71–73

Bennett, M. and Hart, C.A. (1994) Hantavirus infection. *J. Med. Microbiol.,* **41,** 71–73

Bier, J.W. and Sawyer, T.K. (1990) Amoebae isolated from eyewash stations. *Current Microbiol.,* **20,** 349

BMA (1989) *Infection Control,* London, Edward Arnold

BMA (1990) Precautions against tuberculosis. *Br. Med. J.,* **300,** 995

BMA (1995a) *Code of Practice for the Implementation of the UK Hepatitis B Immunisation Guidelines for the Protection of Patients and Staff,* London, British Medical Association

BMA (1995b) *Code of Practice for the Safe Use and Disposal of Sharps,* 2nd edn, London, British Medical Association

Brady, M.T. (1986) Cytomegalovirus infections: occupational risk for health professionals. *Am. J. Infect. Control,* **14,** 197–203

Brandt, F.H., Ware, D.A. and Visvesvara, G.S. (1989) Viability of *Acanthamoeba* cysts in ophthalmic solutions. *Appl. Envir. Microbiol.,* **55,** 1144–1146

British Standards (1990) *BS 7320. Specification for Sharps Containers,* London, British Standards Institution

British Thoracic Society (1990) Control and prevention of tuberculosis in Britain; an update and Code of Practice. *Br. Med. J.,* **300,** 195–220

Brown, C.M., Campbell, I. and Priest, F.G. (1987) *Introduction to Biotechnology,* Oxford, Blackwell Scientific Publications

Buckle, A.E and Saunders, M.F. (1990) An appraisal of bioassay methods for the detection of mycotoxins. *Lett. Appl. Microbiol.,* **10,** 155–160

Buxton, D. (1986) Potential danger to pregnant women of *Chlamydia psittaci* from sheep. *Vet. Rec.,* **118,** 510–511

Calder, I.M. (1987) *Code of health and safety for the funeral service,* Cooperative Funeral Services Managers Association, British Institute of Embalmers, National Association of Funeral Directors, British Institute of Funeral Directors

Carter, S.D. (1992) Cross-infection risks associated with high-speed dental drills. *J. Clin. Microbiol.,* **30,** 1902 (Letter)

Casemore, D.P. (1990) Epidemiological aspects of human cryptosporidiosis. *Epidemiol. Infect.,* **104,** 1–28

CDC (1974) *Classification of Etiologic Agents on the Basis of Hazard,* 4th edn, Atlanta, US Public Health Service

CDC (1993) Update: outbreak of hantavirus infection—south west United States. *Morb. Mort. Wkly Rep.,* **42,** 495–496

CDC (1994) Hantavirus pulmonary syndrome—United States 1993. Centers for Disease Control. *Morb. Mort. Wkly Rep.,* **43,** 45–48

Cieslak, P., Barrett, T.J., Griffin, P.M., *et al.* (1993) *Escherichia coli* infection from a manured garden. *Lancet,* **342,** 367

Collins, C.H. (1983) *Laboratory-Aquired Infections,* 1st edn, London, Butterworth

Collins, C.H. (1993) *Laboratory-Acquired Infections,* 3rd edn, Oxford, Butterworth-Heinemann

Collins, C.H. (1994) *Blood-borne Diseases in the Workplace,* Schenectady, Genium Publishing (Leeds, H. & H. Scientific)

Collins, C.H. and Beale, A.J. (eds) (1992) *Safety in Industrial Microbiology and Biotechnology,* Oxford, Butterworth-Heinemann

Collins, C.H. and Grange, J.M. (1990) *The Microbiological Hazards of Occupations,* Occupational Hygiene Monograph No. 17, Leeds, H. & H. Scientific

Collins, C.H. and Kennedy, D.A. (1988) A review: Microbiological hazards of occupational needlestick and 'sharps' injuries. *J. Appl. Bact.*, **62**, 385–402

Collins C.H. and Kennedy, D.A. (1992) The microbiological hazards of municipal and clinical wastes. *J. Appl. Bact.*, **72**, 1–6

Collins, C.H. and Kennedy, D.A. (1993) *The Treatment and Disposal of Clinical Waste*, Leeds, H. & H. Scientific

Collins, C.H., Grange, J.M. and Yates, M.D. (1984) A review: mycobacteria in water. *J. Appl. Bact.*, **57**, 193–211

Collins, C.H., Grange, J.M., Noble, W.C. and Yates, M.D. (1984) A review: *Mycobacterium marinum* infections in man. *J. Hyg.*, **94**, 135–149

Collins, C.H., Hartley, E.G. and Pilsworth, R. (1974) *The Prevention of Laboratory Acquired Infections*, PHLS Monograph No. 6, London, Public Health Laboratory Service

Collins, C.H., Lyne, P.M. and Grange, J.M. (eds) (1995) *Collins and Lyne's Microbiological Methods*, 7th edn, Oxford, Butterworth-Heinemann

Cossar, J.H., Reid, D., Grist, N.R., Fallon, R.J., *et al.* (1985) Illness associated with travel. *Travel Med. Int.*, **3**, 13–18

Coralli, C.H. (1985) Promoting health in international travel. *Nurse Pract.*, **10**, 28–43

Crawford, G.R and Grant, Y. (1994) Legionella in potting soils. *Br. J. Biomed. Sci.*, **51**, 375–376

Crook, B. (1991) Spore wars. *Lab. Pract.*, **41**, 19–23

Crook, B. (1992) Microbe-containing oil mists—a respiratory hazard? *Occup. Hlth Rev.*, Feb/Mar, 1991, 24–26

Crook, B. (1994) Aerobiological investigation of occupational allergy in agriculture in the UK. *Grana*, **33**, 81–84

Crook, B. (1995) Inertial samplers: biological perspectives. In: *Bioaerosols Handbook* (eds C.S. Cox and C.A. Wathes), London, Lewis, pp. 247–264

Crook, B. and Lacey, J. (1988) Enumeration of airborne microorganisms in work environments. *Envir. Tech. Lett.*, **9**, 515–520

Crook, B. and Lacey, J. (1991) Airborne allergenic microorganisms associated with mushroom cultivation. *Grana*, **30**, 446–449

Crook, B., Higgins, S. and Lacey, J. (1987), Airborne Gram-negative bacteria associated with the handling of domestic waste. In: *Advances in Aerobiology* (eds G. Boehm and R.M. Leuschner), Basel, Birkhäuser Verlag, pp. 371–375

Crook, B., Robertson, J.F., Travers Glass, S.D.A., Boothroyd, E.M., *et al.* (1991) Airborne dust, ammonia, microorganisms and antigens in pig confinement houses and the respiratory health of exposed farm workers. *Am. Ind. Hyg. Assoc. J.*, **52**, 271–279

Crook, B., Venables K.M. Lacey, J. and Musk A.W. (1988) Dust exposure and respiratory symptoms in a UK bakery. In *Aerosols: their Generation, Behaviour and Application*, (ed. W.D. Griffiths) London, The Aerosol Society, pp. 341–345

Cutler, S.J. and Wright, D.J.M. (1994) Predictive value of serology in diagnosing Lyme borreliosis. *J. Clin. Pathol.*, **47**, 344–349

Dancer, S.J. (1991) A hospital outbreak of infection with *Bacillus* spp. associated with a building site. *J. Med. Microbiol.*, **34**, v (abstract)

Danham, K.J. (1985) Zoonotic diseases of occupational significance in agriculture. *Int. J. Zoonoses*, **121**, 163–191

Departments of Environment and Health (1990) *Cryptosporidiosis in Water Supplies*, Report of the Group of Experts, London, HMSO, 230 pp

de Week, A.L., Gutersohn, J. and Butikofer, E. (1969) La maladie des laveurs (Käserwasserk-rankheit): une forme particulière du syndrom—poumon de fermier. *Schweiz. med. Wschr.*, **99**, 872–876

Dewhurst, A.C., Cooper M.J. Kahn, S.M., Pallet, A.P., *et al.* (1990) Aspergillosis in immuno-suppressed patients; potential hazard of building work. *Br. Med. J.*, **301**, 802–804

do Pico, G.A. (1986) Report on diseases. *Am. J. Ind. Med.*, **10**, 261–265

Doyle, L., Gallagher, K., Heath, B.S. and Patterson, W.B. (1989) An outbreak of infectious conjunctivitis spread by microscopes. *J. Occup. Med.*, **31**, 758–762

Duffus, J.H. and Brown, L.M. (1985) Health aspects of biotechnology. *Ann. Occup. Hyg.*, **29**, 1–12

European Commission (1976) *Council Directive Relating to the Quality of Bathing Water*, 76/160/EEC, Brussels

European Commission (1980) *Council Directive Relating to the Quality of Drinking Water*, 80/78/EEC, Brussels

European Commission (1990) *Council Directive on the Protection of Workers from Risks Related to Exposure to Biological Agents at Work*, 90/677/EEC, Brussels

European Commission (1992) *Council Directive on Pregnant Workers*, 92/85/EEC, Brussels

Ferguson, I.R. (1991) Leptospirosis update. *Br. Med. J.*, **302**, 128–129

Ferguson, I.R. (1993) Rats, fish and Weil's disease. *Safety Hlth Pract.*, December 1993, 12–15

Fink, J. (1986) Hypersensitivity pneumonitis. In *Occupational Respiratory Disease* (ed. J.A. Merchant *et al.*), Washington, US Department of Health and Human Welfare, pp. 481–500

Finnegan, M.J., Pickering C.A.C. and Burge, P.S. (1984) The sick building syndrome: prevalence studies. *Br. Med. J.*, **289**, 1573–1575

Flannigan, B. (1987) Mycotoxins in the air. *Int. Biodet.*, **23**, 73–78

Flannigan, B., McCabe, E. and McGarry, F. (1991) Allergenic and toxigenic microorganisms in houses. *J. Appl. Bact. Symp.* Supplement, No. 20, 61S–73S

Flewett, T.H. (1980) Safety in the virology laboratory. In *Recent Advances in Clinical Virology* 2 (ed. A.P. Waterson), Edinburgh, Churchill Livingstone, pp. 169–187

Forster, H.W., Crook, B., Platts, B.W., Lacey, J., *et al.* (1989) Investigation of organic aerosols generated during sugar beet slicing. *Am. Ind. Hyg. Assoc. J.*, **50**, 44–50

Francis, D.P., Holmes, M.A. and Brandon, G. (1975) *Pasteurella multocida* infections after domestic animal bites and scratches. *J. Am. Med. Assoc.*, **233**, 42–45

French, J.C., Messinger, H.B. and McCarthy, J.A. (1970) A study of *Toxoplasma gondii* infection in farm and non-farm groups in the same geographical location. *Am. J. Epidemiol.*, **91**, 185–191

Frommer, W. and a Working Party of the European Federation of Biotechnology. (1989) Safe biotechnology 3. Safety precautions for handling microorganisms of different risk classes. *Appl. Microbiol. Biotechnol.*, **30**, 541–552

Frommer, W. and a Working Party of the European Federation of Biotechnology. (1992) Safe biotechnology 4. Recommendations for safety levels for biotechnological operations with microorganism that cause diseases of plants. *Appl. Microbiol. Biotechnol.*, **38**, 139–140

Frommer, W. and a Working Party of the European Federation of Biotechnology. (1993) Safe biotechnology 5. Recommendations for safe work with human and animal cell cultures concerning potential human pathogens. *Appl. Microbiol. Biotechnol.*, **39**, 141–147

Georghiou, P. (1980) Mycobacterium as an occupational hazard in abattoir workers. *Aust. NZ. J. Med.*, **19**, 409

Gestal, J.J. (1987) Occupational hazards in hospitals: risk of infection. *Br. J. Ind. Med.*, **44**, 435–442

Gittins, M.J. (1989) Hazards of the working environment. *Safety Pract.*, **7**, 8–11

Glass, D.C. (ed.) (1989) *Proceedings of a Conference on the health hazards of cutting oils and their control*, Birmingham, University of Birmingham

Goldberg, D.J., Wrench, J.G., Collier, P.W., Emslie, J.A.N., *et al.* (1989) Lochgoilhead fever: outbreak of non-pneumonic legionellosis due to *Legionella micdadei*. *Lancet*, **1**, 316–318

Goodley, J.M., Clayton, Y.M. and Hay, J. (1993) Environmental sampling for aspergilli during building construction on a hospital site. *J. Hosp. Infect.*, **26**, 27–35

Gorbey, G.L. and Peacock, J.E. (1988) *Erysipelothrix rhusiopathiae* endocarditis: microbiologic, epidemiologic and clinical features of an occupational disease. *Rev. Infect. Dis.*, **10**, 317–325

Greene, J.J. and Bannan, L.T. (1985) Potato riddlers' lung. *Irish Med. J.*, **78**, 282–284

Grist N. (1988) Hantaviruses are here in Scotland. *J. Infect. Dis.*, **17**, 83–87

Grist N. and Emslie, J. (1991) Infections in British clinical laboratories, 1988–9. *J. Clin. Pathol.*, **44**, 667–681

Gröschel, D.H.M. (1980) Air sampling in hospitals. *Ann. N.Y. Acad. Sci.*, **353**, 230–240

Hagman, L. (1990) Health effects of exposure to endotoxins and organic dust in poultry slaughterhouse workers. *Int. Arch. Occup. Environ. Hlth*, **62**, 159–163

Hambleton, P, Bennett, A.M. and Leaver, G. (1992) Biosafety monitoring devices for biotechnology processes. *Trends in Biotech.*, **10**, 192–199

Harrington, J.A., Gill, F.S., Aw, T-C., *et al.* (1992) *Pocket Consultant in Occupational Health*, 3rd edn, Oxford, Blackwell Scientific Publications

Hay, R.J., Clayton, Y.M. and Goodley, J.M. (1995) Fungal aerobiology: how, when and where? *J. Hosp. Inf.*, **30** (Supplement), 352–357

Healing, T.D., Hoffman, P.N. and Young, S.E.J. (1995) The infection hazards of human cadavers. *CDR Review*, 5, Review No. 5, R61–R68

Heap, B.J. and McCullough, M.L.B. (1991) Giardiasis and occupational risk in sewage workers. *Lancet*, **338**, 1152

Heptonstall, J., Gill, O.N., Porter, K., Black, M.B., *et al.* (1993) Health-care workers and HIV; surveillance of occupationally-acquired infection in the United Kingdom. *Comm. Dis. Rep.*, **3**, R147–R152

Hruszkewycz, V., Ruben, B., Hypes, C., Bostic G.D., *et al.* (1992) A cluster of pseudo-fungaemia associated with hospital renovation adjacent to the microbiology laboratory. *Infect. Control Hosp. Epidem.*, **13**, 147–150

HSE (1979) *Anthrax: health hazards*, EH23

HSE (1984) *Categorization of pathogens according to hazard and categories of containment*, Advisory Committee on Dangerous Pathogens

HSE (1986) *Guide to the Reporting of Injuries, Diseases and Dangerous Occurrences Regulations 1985*, HS(R)23 (see also Appendix 2)

HSE (1989) *Precautions against humidifier fever in the print industry*, IAC/L28

HSE (1990a) *What you should know about allergy laboratory animals*

HSE (1990b) *Categorization of pathogens according to hazard and categories of containment*, 2nd edn, Advisory Committee on Dangerous Pathogens

HSE (1991a) *The prevention and control of legionellosis (including legionnaires' disease)*, Approved Code of Practice, L8

HSE (1991b) *Safety in health service laboratories. Safe working and the prevention of infection in clinical laboratories*

HSE (1991c) *Safety in health service laboratories. Safe working and the prevention of infection in the mortuary and post-mortem room*

HSE (1991d) *Safety in health service laboratories. Safe working and the prevention of infection in clinical laboratories—model rules for staff and visitors*

HSE (1992a) *Metalworking fluids—health precautions*, EH62

HSE (1992b) *Health and safety in animal facilities*

HSE (1992c) *Management of Health and Safety at Work. Approved Code of Practice*, L21

HSE (1993a) *Grain dust*, EH66

HSE (1993b) *Grain dust in maltings (maximum exposure limits)*, EH67

HSE (1993c) *The occupational zoonoses*

HSE (1993d) *The control of legionellosis including legionnaires' disease*, HS(G)70, 3rd edn

HSE (1993e) *Safe disposal of clinical waste*

HSE (1994a) *Precautions for work with human and animal transmissible spongiform encephalopathies*, Advisory Committee on Dangerous Pathogens

HSE (1994b) *General COSHH (Control of Substances Hazardous to Health)*, Approved Codes of Practice

HSE (1995a) *Categorization of pathogens according to hazard and categories of containment*, 4th edn, Advisory Committee on Dangerous Pathogens

HSE (1995b) *Occupational exposure limits 1994*, EH40/94

Hubbert, W.T. and Rosen, M.N. (1970) *Pasteurella multocida* infections in man unrelated to animal bites. *Am. J. Pub. Hlth*, **60**, 1109–1116

Hunt, D.L. (1995) Human immunodeficiency virus type 1 and other blood-borne pathogens. In *Laboratory Safety. Principles and Practice*, 2nd edn, (eds D.O. Fleming, J. Richardson, J.L. Tullis and D. Vesley), Washington, DC, American Association for Microbiology Press, pp. 33–66

Hunter, P.R. (1991) An introduction to the biology, ecology and potential public health significance of the blue-green algae. *PHLS Microbiology Digest*, **8**, 11–13

Hunter, P.R. (1994) Environmental sampling for aspergilli during building construction on a hospital site. *J. Hosp. Infect.*, **26**, 27–31

IIAC (1993) Industrial Injuries Advisory Council, Periodic Report, London, HMSO

Jeffries, D.J. (1995) Viral hazards to and from health workers. *J. Hosp. Inf.*, **30** (Supplement), 140–155

Johnson, C.L., Bernstein, I.L., Gallagher, J.S., Bonventre, P.F., *et al.* (1980) Familial hypersensitivity pneumonia induced by *Bacillus subtilis*. *Am. Rev. Resp. Dis.*, **122**, 339–348

Jones, E., Remis, R., Tait, K., McGee, H., *et al.* (1982) An outbreak of Pontiac fever related to whirlpool use. Abstracts of the Epidemiological Intelligence Conference, Atlanta, Centers for Disease Control

Kassianos, G.C. (1994) *Immunization—Precautions and Contraindications*, 2nd edn, Oxford, Blackwell

Kaustova, J., Olsovsky, Z., Kubin, M., Zatlovkal, O., *et al.* (1981) Epidemic occurrence of *Mycobacterium kansasii* in water supplies. *J. Hyg. Epidemiol. Microbiol. Immunol.*, **25**, 24–30

Kilvington, S. and White, D.G. (1994) Acanthamoeba: biology, ecology and human disease. *Rev. Med. Microbiol.*, **5**, 12–20

Krasinski, K., Holzman, R.S, Hanna, B. and Greco, M.A. (1985) Nosocomial fungal infection during hospital renovation. *Infect. Control*, **6**, 278–282

Küenzi. M. and a Working Party of the European Federation of Biotechnology. (1985) Safe biotechnology: general considerations. *Appl. Microbiol. Biotechnol.*, **21**, 1–6

Küenzi. M. and a Working Party of the European Federation of Biotechnology. (1987) Safe biotechnology: 2. The classification of microorganisms causing diseases in plants. *Appl. Microbiol. Biotechnol.*, **27**, 105

Lacey, J. (1971) *Thermoactinomyces sacchari*, sp. nov., a thermophilic actinomycete causing bagassosis. *J. Gen. Microbiol.*, **66**, 327–338

Lacey, J. (1980) The microflora of grain dusts. In *Occupational Lung Disorders—Focus on Grain Dusts and Health* (eds J.A. Dosman and D.J. Cotton). London, Academic Press, pp. 417–440

Lacey, J. (1989a) Airborne micro-organisms in the works environment. *Occup. Hlth Rev.* (Feb-March), 1989, 20–21

Lacey, J. (1989b) Airborne hazards from agricultural materials. In *Airborne Deteriogens and Pathogens* (ed. B. Flannigan), Kew, Biodeterioration Society, pp. 13–28

Lacey, J. and Crook, B. (1988) Fungal and actinomycete spores as pollutants of the workplace and occupational allergens. *Ann. Occup. Hyg.* **32**, 515–533

Lacey, J. and Dutkiewicz, J. (1994) Bioaerosols and occupational lung diseases. *J. Aerosol Sci.*, **25**, 1371–1404

Lacey, J., Pepys, J. and Cross, T. (1972) Actinomycete and fungus spores in air as respiratory allergens. In *Safety in Microbiology* (eds D.A. Shapton and R.G. Board), Society for Applied Bacteriology Technical Series No. 6, London, Academic Press, pp. 151–184

Lacey, J., Auger, P., Eduard, W., Norn, S., *et al.* (1994) Tannins and mycotoxins. In *Causative Agents for Organic Dust Related Disease* (eds R. Rylander and Y. Peterson), *Am. J. Ind. Med.*, **25**, 141–144

Lelieveld, H.L.M. and a Working Party of the European Federation of Biotechnology (1995) Safe Biotechnology 6. Safety assessment in respect of human health of microorganism used in biotechnology. *Appl. Microbiol. Biotechnol.*, **43**, 389–393

Lentino, J.R., Rosenkrantz, M.A., Michaels, J.A., Kurup, V.P., *et al.* (1982) Nosocomial aspergillosis. A retrospective review of airborne disease secondary to road construction and contaminated air conditioners. *Am. J. Epidemiol.*, **116**, 430–437

Lewis, D.L. and Boe, R.K. (1992) Cross-infection risks associated with current procedures for using high-speed dental handpieces. *J. Clin. Microbiol.*, **30**, 401–406

Lieberman, D.F., Israeli, E. and Fink, B.S. (1991) Risk assessment of biological hazards in the biotechnology industry. *Occup. Med. State of the Art Reviews*, **6**, 285–299

London Waste Regulation Authority (1994) *Guidelines for the Segregation, Handling, Transport and Disposal of Clinical Waste*, 2nd edn, London

Loriot, J. and Tourte, J. (1990) Hazards of contact lenses used by workers. *Int. Arch. Occup. Environ. Hlth*, **62**, 105–108

McDonald, L. (1989) Blood exposure and protection in funeral homes. *Am. J. Infect. Control*, **17**, 193–195

McLaughlin, J. and Low, J.C. (1994) Primary cutaneous listeriosis in adults: an occupational disease of veterinarians and farmers. *Vet Rec. (Dec.)*, **24/31**, 615–617

Malaty, H.M., Evans, D.J., Abramovitch, K., Evans, D.G. *et al.* (1992) *Helicobacter pylori* infection in dental workers: a seroepidemiological study. *Am. J. Gastroent.*, **87**, 1728–1731

Malmberg, P., Rask Andersen, A., Hogland, S., Kalomodin-Hedman, B. *et al.* (1988) Incidence of organic dust toxic syndrome and allergic alveolitis in Swedish farmers. *Int. Arch. Allergy*, **87**, 47–54

Malone, E. (1994) Leptospirosis—an important zoonosis. *Irish Vet.*, **47**, 272–273

Masterton, R.G. and Green, A.D. (1991) Dissemination of human pathogens by airline travel. In *Pathogens in the Environment*, Society for Applied Bacteriology Symposium Supplement, No 20, pp. 31S–38S

Moss, M. (1989) Mycotoxins of *Aspergillus* and other filamentous fungi. In *Filamentous Fungi in Foods and Feeds*, Society for Applied Bacteriology Symposium Supplement No. 18, pp. 69S–82S

Murray, K., Selleck, P., Hooper, P., *et al.* (1995) A morbilli-virus that caused fatal disease in horses and humans. *Science*, **268**, 94–97

Newman Taylor, A.J. (1994) Occupational asthma. In *Occupational Lung Disorders*, 3rd edn (ed. W.R. Parkes), Oxford, Butterworth-Heinemann, pp. 710–729

Nwanyanwu, O.C. (1989) Exposure to and precautions for blood and body fluids among workers in funeral homes. *Am. J. Infect. Control*, **8**, 208–212

O'Brien, I.M., Bull, J., Creamer, B., Sepulveda, R. *et al.* (1978) Asthma and extrinsic allergic alveolitis due to *Merulius lacrymans*. *Clin. Allergy*, **8**, 535–542

OECD (1986) *Recombinant DNA Safety Considerations*, Paris, Organization for Economic Cooperation and Development

OECD (1992) *Safety Considerations for Biotechnology*, Paris, Organization for Economic Cooperation and Development

Olcerst, R.B. (1987) Microscopes and ocular infections. *Am. Ind. Hyg. Assoc J.*, **48**, 425–431

Oliphant, J.W., Gordon, D.A., Meis, A. and Parker, R.R. (1949) Q fever in laundry workers presumably transmitted from contaminated laundry. *Am. J. Hyg.*, **49**, 76–82

Oliver, P.O. (1979) Medical hazards at sea. *Br. J. Hosp. Med.*, **22**, 615–618

Palchak, R.B., Cohen, R., Ainslie, M. and Hoener, C.L. (1988) Airborne endotoxin associated with industrial scale production of protein products in Gram-negative bacilli. *Am. Ind. Hyg. Assoc. J.*, **49**, 420–421

Parker, S.O.L and Holliman, R.E. (1992) Toxoplasmosis and laboratory workers: a case-control assessment of risk. *Med. Lab. Sci.*, **49**, 103–106

Patel, P., Northfield, T. and Maxwell, D. (1995) Update: *Helicobacter pylori. Gastroenterology in Practice*, Springer, Berlin, 1995

Patterson, W.B., Craven, D.E., Schwartz, D.A., Nardell, E.A. *et al.* (1985) Occupational hazards to hospital personnel. *Ann. Intern. Med.*, **102**, 658–680

Paul, M., Himmelstein, J., Weinstein, S., Pransky, G., *et al.* (1989) Ocular infections and the industrial use of microscopes. *J. Occup. Med.*, **31**, 763–766

Perraud, M., Piens, M.A., Nicoloyannis, N., Girard, P., *et al.* (1987) Invasive nosocomial pulmonary aspergillosis: risk factors and hospital building works. *Epidemiol. Infect.*, **99**, 407–412

Pether, J.V.S., Thurlow, J., Palfreyman, T.G. and Lloyd, G. (1993) Acute hantavirus infection presenting as hypersensitivity vacuolitis with arthropathology. *J. Infect.*, **26**, 75–77

Pickering, C.A. and Newman Taylor, A.J. (1994) Extrinsic allergic bronchioalveolitis (hypersensitivity pneumonia). In *Occupational Lung Disorders* (ed. W.R. Parkes), Oxford, Butterworth-Heinemann, pp. 667–709

Pratt, D.S. and May, J.J. (1984) Feed-associated respiratory illness in farmers. *Arch. Environ. Health*, **39**, 43–48

Ramazzini, B. (1713) *De Morbis Artificum, Diatriba*, translated with notes by W.C. Wright. University of Chicago Press, 1940

Ridley, R.M. and Baker, H.F. (1993) Occupational risk of Creutzfeld–Jakob disease. *Lancet*, **341**, 641–642

Robb, J., Norval, M. and Neill, W.A.Q. (1990) The use of tissue culture for the detection of mycotoxins. *Lett. Appl. Microbiol.*, **10**, 161–165

Roberts, W., Grist, N.R. and Guroud, P. (1967) Humam abortion associated with infection by ovine abortion agent. *Br. Med. J.*, **4**, 37

Robertson, A.S., Weir, D.C. and Burge, P.S. (1988) Occupational asthma due to oil mists. *Thorax*, **43**, 200–205

Royal College of Nursing (1987) *Introduction to Hepatitis B and Nursing Guidelines for Infection Control*, London

Royal Institute of Public Health and Hygiene (1995) *Handbook of Mortuary Practice and Safety*, London

Rylander, R. (1981) Bacterial toxins and the etiology of byssinosis. *Chest*, **79**, 38s–43s

Rylander, R. (1986) Lung diseases caused by organic dusts in the farm environment. *Am. J. Ind. Med.*, **10**, 221–227

Rylander, R. and Haglind, P. (1984) Airborne endotoxins and humidifier fever. *Clin. Allergy*, **14**, 109–112

Rylander, R., Lundholm, M. and Clark, C.S. (1983) Exposure to aerosols of microorganisms and toxins during handling of sewage sludge. In *Biological Health Risk of Sludge Disposal to Land in Cold Climates* (eds P.M. Wallis and D.L. Lohmann), Calgary, University of Calgary Press, pp. 69–78

Rylander, R., Haglind, P., Lundholm, M., Maltsby, M. *et al.* (1978) Humidifier fever and endotoxin exposure. *Clin. Allergy*, **8**, 511–516

Rylander, R., Anderssen, K., Belin, L., Beglund, D. *et al.* (1976) Sewage workers' syndrome. *Lancet*, **2**, 478–479

Salkinoja-Salonen, M.S., Helander, I. and Rylander, R. (1982) Toxic bacterial dusts associated with plants. In *Bacteria and Plants* (eds M. Rhodes-Roberts and F.A. Skinner), Society for Applied Bacteriology Technical Series 10, London, Academic Press, pp. 219–233

Sawcer, S.J., Yuill, G.M., Esmonde, T.F.G., *et al.* (1993) Creutzfeldt–Jacob disease in an individual occupationally exposed to BSE. *Lancet*, **341**, 642

Sepkowitz, K.A. (1994) Tuberculosis and the health care worker: a historical perspective. *Ann. Intern. Med.*, **120**, 71–79

Shakespeare, A.T. and Poole, C.J.M. (1993) Sewage workers and hepatitis *Am. Occup. Hlth*, **45**, 364–366

Shanson, D.C. (1988) *Microbiology in Clinical Practice*, 2nd edn (revised), Oxford, Butterworth-Heinemann

Sharp, J.C.M. (1993) Infections in sport. In *Essentials of Sport Medicine*, 2nd edn (ed. G. R. McLatchie), London, Churchill–Livingstone, pp. 112–125

Sharp, J.C.M. (1994) Infections in sport. *Br. Med. J.*, **308**, 1702–1706

Sharp, J.C.M. and Adams, E.I. (1990) Scrumpox. *Comm. Dis Scotland, Weekly Report 24*, No. 17, 7–8

Shi, Z.C. and Lei, P.C. (1986) Occupational mycoses. *Br. J. Ind. Med.*, **43**, 500–501

Shute, P., Jeffries. D.J. and Maddocks, A.C. (1979) Scrumpox caused by herpes simplex virus. *Br. Med. J.*, **2**, 1629

Skidmore, S.J. (1995) Hepatitis E. *Br. Med. J.*, **310**, 414–415

Sorenson, W.G. (1989) Health impact of mycotoxins in the home and workplace. In *Biodeterioration Research 2* (eds G.C. Llewellyn and E.C. O'Rear), Oxford, Pergamon Press, pp. 201–215

Thomas, P.D. and Joynson, D.H.M. (1994) Occupational infections of agricultural workers. *PHLS Microbiology Digest*, **11**, 206–210

Timothy, E.M. and Mepham, P. (1984) Outbreak of infectious hepatitis among sewage sludge spreaders. *Comm. Dis. Rep.*, **3**, 3

Tobie, J.E. and McCullough, N.B (1961) Infections in meat inspectors. *J. Am. Vet. Med. Assoc.*, **138**, 434–436

Tompkins, D.C. and Steigbigel, R.T. (1993) Rochalimea's role in cat scratch fever and bacillary angiomatosis. *Ann. Int. Med.*, **118**, 388–390

Tookey, P. and Peckham, C.S. (1991) Does cytomegalovirus present an occupational risk? *Arch. Dis. Child.*, **66**, 1009–1010

Tookey, P. and Logan, S. (1994) Occupational risk of cytomegalovirus. *Rev. Med. Microbiol.*, **5**, 33–38

Travers Glass, S.A., Griffin, P. and Crook, B. (1989) Microbial contamination of oil mists in engineering works. *Biodeterioriation Society Occasional Publication, No 6* (ed. B. Flannigan), London, The Biodeterioration Society, pp. 69–73

Travers Glass, S.A, Griffin, P. and Crook, B. (1991) Bacterially contaminated oil mists in engineering works; a possible respiratory hazard. *Grana*, **30**, 404–406

Tuijnenberg-Muijs, G. (1992) Monitoring and validation in biotechnological processes. In *Safety in Industrial Microbiology and Biotechnology* (eds C.H. Collins and A.J. Beale), Oxford, Butterworth-Heinemann, pp. 214–238

Tyler, J. (1985) Occurrence in water of viruses of public health significance. Society for Applied Bacteriology Symposium Supplement No. 14, pp. 37S–46S

Tyndall, R.L. (1987) The presence of free-living amoebae in portable and stationary eye wash stations. *Am. Indust. Hyg. Assoc. J.,* **48**, 933–934

UK Health Departments (1978) *Code of Practice for the Prevention of Infection in Clinical Laboratories and Post-mortem rooms,* London, HMSO

UK Health Departments (1981) *Report of the Advisory Group on the management of patients with with spongiform encephalopathy [Creutzfeldt–Jacob Disease (CJD)] to the Chief Medical Officers,* Departmental Advice Note DA(81)22, London, HMSO

UK Health Departments (1988a) *The Control of Legionellae in Health Care Premises. A Code of Practice,* London, HMSO

UK Health Departments (1988b) *Information to undertakers—infectious diseases,* PL/CMO/88/8

UK Health Departments (1990a) *Guidance for Clinical Health Care Workers: Protection against Infections with HIV and Hepatitis Viruses,* London, HMSO

UK Health Departments (1990b) Control of tuberculosis in NHS employees. Executive letter, EH(90) 174

UK Health Departments (1992) *Immunization against Infectious Diseases,* London, HMSO

UK Health Departments (1993) *Protecting Health Care Workers and Patients from Hepatitis B,* London, Health Publications Unit

Ulfig, K. and Korcz, M. (1983) Isolation of keratinophilic fungi from sewage sludge. *Sabouraudia,* **21**, 247–250

Ulfig, K. and Ulfig, A. (1990) Keratinophilic fungi in bottom sediments of surface waters. *J. Med. Vet. Mycol.,* **28**, 419–422

Viral Hepatitis Prevention Board (1993) *Eliminating Hepatitis B as an Occupational Hazard,* London

Waldron, H.A. (1990) *Lecture Notes on Occupational Medicine,* 4th edn, Oxford, Blackwell Scientific Publications

West, P.A. (1991) Human pathogenic viruses and parasites; emerging parasites in the water cycle. In *Pathogens in the Environment,* Society for Applied Bacteriology Symposium Supplement No. 20, pp. 107S–114S

West, P.A. and Locke, R. (1990) Occupational risks from infectious diseases in the water industry. *J. Inst. Water Environ. Mangt.,* **4**, 520–523

WHO (1979) Safety measures in microbiology. Minimum standards for laboratory safety. *Wld Hlth Org. Wkly Epid. Rec. No. 40,* pp. 340–342

WHO (1982a) *Summary Report of the Working Group on the Health Implications of Biotechnology,* Geneva, World Health Organization

WHO (1982b) *Guidelines for the Control of Leptospirosis,* WHO Offset Publication No 67, Geneva, World Health Organization

WHO (1988) *Guidelines for the Development of a National AIDS Prevention and Control Programme,* WHO AIDS Series No.1, Geneva, World Health Organization

WHO (1989) *Monitoring of National AIDS Prevention and Control Programmes: Guiding Principles,* WHO AIDS Series No.4, Geneva, World Health Organization

WHO (1993) *Laboratory Biosafety Manual,* 2nd edn, Geneva, World Health Organization

WHO (1995) *Biosafety Guidelines for the Production of Vaccines and Biological Products for Medical Use,* Geneva, World Health Organization

Winkler, K.C. and Park, J.A.C. (1992) Assessment of risk. In *Safety in Industrial Microbiology and Biotechnology* (eds C.H. Collins and A.J. Beale), Oxford, Butterworth-Heinemann, pp. 34–74

Woodhead, M. (1994) Infectious diseases and zoonoses. In *Occupational Lung Disorders* (ed. W.R. Parkes), London, Butterworth-Heinemann, pp. 755–777

Index

(The letter 't' indicates a table.)